The Foundation Programme at a Glance

Stuart Carney

MPH MRCPsych FAcadMEd
Dean of Medical Education
King's College London
Guy's Campus
London
Deputy National Director
UK Foundation Programme Office
Cardiff

Derek Gallen

MMed FRCGP FAcadMEd FHEA FRCPE
Postgraduate Dean for Wales
Cardiff University
Cardiff
National Director
UK Foundation Programme Office
Cardiff

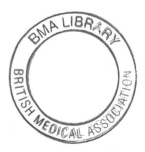
WILEY Blackwell

This edition first published 2014 © 2014 by John Wiley & Sons, Ltd.

Registered office: John Wiley & Sons, Ltd, The Atrium, Southern Gate, Chichester,
West Sussex, PO19 8SQ, UK

Editorial offices: 9600 Garsington Road, Oxford, OX4 2DQ, UK
The Atrium, Southern Gate, Chichester, West Sussex, PO19 8SQ, UK
111 River Street, Hoboken, NJ 07030-5774, USA

For details of our global editorial offices, for customer services and for information about how to apply for
permission to reuse the copyright material in this book please see our website at
www.wiley.com/wiley-blackwell

Library of Congress Cataloging-in-Publication Data

Carney, Stuart, author.
  The Foundation Programme at a glance / Stuart Carney, Derek Gallen.
    p. ; cm. – (At a glance series)
  Includes bibliographical references and index.
  ISBN 978-0-470-65737-9 (pbk. : alk. paper) – ISBN 978-1-118-73459-9 –
ISBN 978-1-118-73460-5 – ISBN 978-1-118-73461-2 (emobi) – ISBN 978-1-118-73462-9 (epdf) – ISBN
978-1-118-73463-6 (epub)
  I. Gallen, Derek, author.   II. Title.   III. Series: At a glance series (Oxford, England)
  [DNLM: 1. Foundation Programme (Great Britain. National Health Service)   2. Clinical
Medicine–methods–Great Britain.   3. Medical Staff, Hospital–education–Great Britain.
4. Inservice Training–methods–Great Britain.   5. National Health Programs–organization &
administration–Great Britain.   WX 203]
  RA972
  362.11068′3–dc23
                                                                          2013024793

A catalogue record for this book is available from the British Library.

Wiley also publishes its books in a variety of electronic formats. Some content that appears in print may not be
available in electronic books.

Cover image: iStockphoto © Sturti
Cover design by Meaden Creative

Set in 9/11.5pt Times by Aptara® Inc., New Delhi, India
Printed and bound in Malaysia by Vivar Printing Sdn Bhd

1   2014

Contents

List of contributors

Anthony Bateman
FRCA
Consultant in Critical Care and Long Term Ventilation
ICU, Western General Hospital
Edinburgh, UK
Chapters 40, 41

Rhodri G. Birtchnell
MBBCh BSc (Hons) FCARCSI
Anaesthetic Registrar
Royal Gwent Hospital
Newport, UK
Chapter 33

Sue Carr
MB BS MMedSci MD FRCP
Consultant Nephrologist/Visiting Professor of Medical Education
Associate Medical Director
University Hospitals of Leicester
Leicester, UK
Chapters 23, 42, 43, 44

Gordon French
FRCA FFICM MBA
Consultant Anaesthetist
Department of Anaesthesia and Critical Care
Northampton General Hospital
Northampton, UK
Chapter 28

Alice Gallen
BSc MBBS
GP Registrar
Nevill Hall Hospital
Abergavenny, UK
Chapter 1

Peter Henriksen
PhD FRCP
Consultant Cardiologist
Edinburgh Heart Centre
Edinburgh, UK
Chapter 39

Patricia Hooper
MBChB BSc MRCP
Specialty Registrar, Gastroenterology
University Hospitals of Leicester NHS Trust
Leicester, UK
Chapters 47, 48

Helen L. Jewitt
MBBCh FRCA
Consultant Anaesthetist
Royal Gwent Hospital
Newport, UK
Chapter 32

Melanie J. T. Jones
MB BCh FRCA MA
Associate Dean for Careers and LTFT Training, Wales
Retired Consultant Anaesthetist
Chapters 5, 6, 31, 32, 33

M. Sian Lewis
MB BCh FRCP FRCPath PCME MBA
Consultant Haematologist Hywel Dda Health Board
Carmarthen, UK
Chapter 24

Laura McGregor
MBChB MRCP (UK) (Rheumatology)
Consultant Rheumatologist
Glasgow Royal Infirmary
Glasgow, UK
Chapter 49

Scott W. Oliver
MBChB BSc (MedSci) (Hons) MRCP (UK) MFMLM
Specialty Registrar, Nephrology and General (Internal)
    Medicine
NHS Lanarkshire
Glasgow, UK
Chapters 19, 21, 25

Matt Outram
FRCA FFICM
Consultant Anaesthetist
Department of Anaesthesia and Critical Care
Northampton General Hospital
Northampton, UK
Chapter 28

Helen A. Padfield
MBBCh FRCA
Specialty Registrar, Anaesthetics
University Hospital of Wales
Cardiff, UK
Chapter 31

Michael D. Page
MD FRCP
Consultant Physician
Royal Glamorgan Hospital
Ynysmaersdy, LLantrisant
Pontyclun, UK
Chapters 45 and 46

Heather Payne
MRCPCH FHEA IHSM
Welsh Government
Cathys Park
Cardiff, UK
Chapters 60, 61, 62, 63

Andrew Steel
FRCP
Consultant Physician
Kettering General Hospital NHS Foundation Trust
Kettering, UK
Chapters 47, 48

Peter S. Topham
MB ChB MD FRCP
Consultant Nephrologist
John Walls Renal Unit
University Hospitals of Leicester
Leicester, UK
Chapters 43 and 44

Rachael Westacott
MB ChB BSci FRCP
Consultant Nephrologist
John Walls Renal Unit
University Hospitals of Leicester
Leicester, UK
Chapters 23, 42, 43, 44

Preface

The 2-year foundation programme was introduced in 2005. Bridging the gap between medical school and specialty training, the original focus of the foundation programme was the assessment and management of the acutely ill patient in a variety of settings. The curriculum has gone through three revisions since the start of the programme and this book encompasses the latest developments. While there continues to be a high emphasis on the management of the acutely ill patient there is now greater emphasis on caring for the 'whole patient' including long-term physical and mental illness. This is a reflection of the needs of the National Health Service (NHS) with a growing elderly population who often have co-morbidities. It is therefore essential that all doctors have a knowledge and understanding of the management of both acute and long-term conditions.

The 'At A Glance' series does not seek to give a comprehensive, in-depth review of each clinical topic or subject but rather a synthesis of the key facts, including the assessment and management of patients with common conditions. The object of this book is to cover the important topics in an easy-to-read and view format. It can be used as an aide-memoir before starting a new placement or to refresh your knowledge before seeing patients with particular clinical problems. It summarizes how to identify, examine, investigate and begin to treat patients. The book also contains valuable information on making the transition from medical school to employment and preparing for specialty training. Topics include time management, dealing with colleagues and communication skills to help in your day-to-day working practice. Top tips are included in all chapters and serve as a quick reference to help ensure you think through the main issues in every case.

This book is primarily aimed at foundation doctors but will also be of benefit to final year medical students As the final year of medical school is mainly spent on the wards dealing with patients, the contents of this book will be very relevant. Educational supervisors may also wish to make reference to the guide as it covers all the key topics in the Foundation Programme Curriculum.

The foundation programme is the start of your career in the NHS and helps you build the confidence and capabilities required to safely and effectively care for patients and progress through to specialty training. We hope you find this book a useful resource in your day-to-day interactions with patients and colleagues alike.

Stuart Carney is the Dean of Medical Education at King's College London and Deputy National Director of the UK Foundation Programme Office. Since 2004 Stuart has been involved in setting up and coordinating the delivery of the foundation programme across the UK. As a psychiatrist and an academic, he has been particularly interested in how the foundation programme prepares graduates to begin to care for the whole patient.

Derek Gallen is the National Director of the UK Foundation Programme Office. He is also the Postgraduate Dean for Wales and Chair of the Conference of Postgraduate Deans UK. He set up the Foundation Programme Office in 2007 in Cardiff and has principally been involved in the recruitment and selection into the 2-year foundation programme. His main interest is in the establishment and development of innovative academic foundation placements.

Acknowledgements

We would like to thank Helen Harvey for all her help and support in getting this manuscript into print. We would also like to thank all the authors of the chapters for their hard work and support.

Finally, we would like to thank our families, Terence, Mary, Paula, Alice, Tom, Rachael, Johny, Luke and particularly Violet Alice Campbell.

Stuart Carney, London
Derek Gallen, Cardiff

The editors would also like to acknowledge the use of part or all of the following chapters from previously published *At a Glance* titles.

Bulstrode, C and Swales, C. *Rheumatology, Orthopaedics and Trauma at a Glance*, 2e. John Wiley & Sons Ltd, 2012
48 Fractures and Dislocations

Davey, P. *Medicine at a Glance*, 3e. Blackwell Publishing Ltd, 2010
61 Acute Visual Impairment: Peggy Frith
78 Coma: David Sprigings

90 Pulmonary Embolism: Keith Channon
104 Asthma: Mark Juniper
105 COPD: Mark Juniper
134 Nutrition: Jeremy Shearman
193 Palliative Care: Jeremy Steele and Laura Tookman
200 Meningitis: Kevin Talbot

Hughes, T and Cruickshank, J. *Adult Emergency Medicine at a Glance*. John Wiley & Sons Ltd, 2011.
42 Stroke
43 Seizures

Katona, C., Cooper, C and Robertson, M. *Psychiatry at a Glance*, 5e. Blackwell Publishing Ltd, 2012.
11 Anxiety disorders

Ward, J and Leach, R. *Respiratory System at a Glance*, 3e. Blackwell Publishing Ltd, 2010.
25 Asthma
26 COPD
35 Pneumothorax
36 Community-acquired pneumonia

List of abbreviations

A&E	accident and emergency		**CV**	curriculum vitae
AAA	abdominal aortic aneurysm		**CVA**	cerebrovascular accident
ABCD	airway, breathing, circulation, disability		**CVP**	central venous pressure
ABG	arterial blood gas		**CVS**	cardiovascular system
ABI	absolute benefit increase		**CXR**	chest X-ray
ABV	alcohol by volume		**D&V**	diarrhoea and vomiting
ACE	angiotensin-converting enzyme		**DBP**	diastolic blood pressure
ACEi	angiotensin-converting enzyme inhibitors		**DEXA**	duel-energy X-ray absorptiometry
ADH	antidiuretic hormone		**DKA**	diabetic ketoacidosis
AF	atrial fibrillation		**DM**	diabetes mellitus
AION	anterior ischaemic optic neuropathy		**DNACPR**	do not attempt cardiopulmonary resuscitation
AKI	acute kidney injury		**DOB**	date of birth
ALS	Advanced Life Support		**DOPS**	direct observation of procedural skills
ANA	antinuclear antibody		**DSM**	Diagnostic Statistical Manual
ANCA	antineutrophil cytoplasmic antibody		**DVT**	deep venous thrombosis
APTT	activated partial thromboplastin time		**EBM**	evidence-based medicine
ARB	angiotensin receptor blocker		**ECF**	extracellular fluid
ARCP	Annual Review of Competence Progression		**ECG**	electrocardiogram
ARR	absolute risk reduction		**ECT**	electroconvulsive therapy
ASO	antistreptolysin O		**EEG**	electroencephalograph
ATS	American Thoracic Society		**EER**	experimental event risk
AUDIT	Alcohol Use Disorder Identification Test		**eGFR**	estimated GFR
AVN	avascular necrosis		**ENT**	ear, nose and throat
AVNRT	atrioventricular node-dependent re-entrant tachycardia		**ESR**	erythrocyte sedimentation rate
AVPU	alert, voice, pain, unresponsive		**EWS**	early warning score
AVRT	atrioventricular re-entrant tachycardia		**F1**	foundation year 1
BMJ	*British Medical Journal*		**F2**	foundation year 2
BNF	*British National Formulary*		**FACD**	foundation achievement of competence document
BP	blood pressure		**FAIR**	feedback, activity, individualize, relevant
BPF	bronchopleural fistula		**FAST**	face, arm, speech, time to call ambulance
bpm	beats per minute		**FAST**	focussed assessment with sonography for trauma
BRVO	branch retinal vein occlusion		**FBC**	full blood count
BTS	British Thoracic Society		**FEV$_1$**	forced expiratory volume in 1 second
CAP	community-acquired pneumonia		**FFP**	fresh frozen plasma
CBD	case-based discussion		**FP**	foundation programme
CBT	cognitive behavioural therapy		**FSD**	foundation school director
CCF	congestive cardiac failure		**FSM**	foundation school manager
CCTR	Cochrane Controlled Trials Register		**FTPD/T**	foundation training programme director/tutor
CI	confidence interval		**FVC**	forced vital capacity
CK	creatinine kinase		**GABA**	gamma-aminobutyric acid
CKD	chronic kidney disease		**GAD**	generalized anxiety disorder
CNS	central nervous system		**GCS**	Glasgow Coma Scale
CO	cardiac output		**GFR**	glomerular filtration rate
CO$_2$	carbon dioxide		**GH**	growth hormone
COPD	chronic obstructive pulmonary disease		**GI**	gastrointestinal
CPAP	continuous positive airway pressure		**GMC**	General Medical Council
CPM	central pontine myelinolysis		**GORD**	gastroesophageal reflux disease
CPPD	calcium pyrophosphate dihydrate disease		**GP**	general practitioner
CPR	cardiopulmonary resuscitation		**GU**	genito-urinary
Cr	creatinine		**Hb**	haemoglobin
CRP	C-reactive protein		**HDU**	high dependency unit
CRT	capillary refill time		**HHT**	hereditary haemorrhagic telangiectasia
CRVO	central retinal vein occlusion		**HIV**	human immunodeficiency virus
CSF	cerebrospinal fluid		**HLA**	human leukocyte antigen
CT	computed tomography		**HOCM**	hypertrophic obstructive cardiomyopathy

HR	heart rate	PION	posterior ischaemic optic neuropathy
IBD	irritable bowel disease	pMDI	paediatric metered dose inhaler
ICD	International Classification of Diseases	PR	per rectum
IgE	immunoglobulin E	PSP	primary spontaneous pneumothorax
IGF	intraglomerular filtration	RAAMbo	represent, allocation, account, measurement (blind, objective)
IHD	ischaemic heart disease		
IMCA	Independent Mental Capacity Advocate/Advisor	RBI	relative benefit increase
INR	international normalized ratio	RCT	randomized controlled trial
IPA	inflammatory polyarthritis	RDS	respiratory distress syndrome
IPT	interpersonal therapy	RR	respiratory rate /risk ratio
ITU	intensive treatment unit	RRR	relative risk reduction
IUCD	intrauterine contraceptive device	RV	residual volume
IV	intravenous	SAH	subarachnoid haemorrhage
IVDU	intravenous drug use	SaO_2	arterial oxygen saturation
ivi	intravenous insulin	SARS	severe acute respiratory syndrome
JVP	jugular venous pressure	SBP	systolic blood pressure
LFT	liver function test	SCr	serum creatinine
LMW	low molecular weight	SIADH	syndrome of inappropriate ADH
LP	lumbar puncture	SIGN	Scottish Inter-Collegiate Guideline Network
LRT	lower respiratory tract	SIRS	systemic inflammatory response syndrome
LTFT	less than full time	SLE	supervised learning event
LTOT	long-term oxygen therapy	SNRIs	serotonin noradrenaline re-uptake inhibitors
LV	left ventricle	SOAP	subjective assessment, objective measurement, assessment, plan
LVH	left ventricular hypertrophy		
MAP	mean arterial pressure	SP	secondary pneumothorax
MCCD	Medical Certificate of the Cause of Death	SPO_2	oxygen saturation
MCQ	multiple choice questions	SR	systematic review
MHRA	Medicines and Healthcare Products Regulatory Agency	SRH	stigmata of recent hemorrhage
MI	myocardial infarction	SSRI	selective serotonin re-uptake inhibitor
Mini-CEX	mini clinical evaluation exercise	ST	stroke volume
MRI	magnetic resonance imaging	SV	stroke volume
MRSA	methicillin-resistant *Staphylococcus aureus*	SvO_2	venous oxygen saturation
MSU	mid-stream urine	SVR	systemic vascular resistance
N saline	normal saline	TAB	team assessment of behaviour
NBM	nil by mouth	TB	tubercle bacillus
NES	NHS Education Scotland	TC	total lung capacity
NG	nasogastric	tds	*ter die sumendum* (three times a day)
NHS	National Health Service	TIA	transient ischaemic attack
NICE	National Institute for Health and Care Excellence	tPA	tissue plasminogen activator
NMDA	*N*-methyl-D-aspartate	U&E	urea and electrolytes
NNT	number needed to treat	UO	urine output
NSAID	non-steroidal anti-inflammatory drug	URTI	upper respiratory tract infection
NSPCC	National Society for the Prevention of Cruelty to Children	USS	ultrasound scan
		UTI	urinary tract infection
NSTEMI	non-ST segment elevation myocardial infarction	VF	ventricular fibrillation
OD	overdose	VT	ventricular tachycardia
β-OHB	beta-hydroxybutyrate	WCC	white cell count
ORS	oral rehydration solution	WHO	World Health Organization
PACS	picture archiving and communications system		
PaO_2	arterial partial pressure of oxygen		
PCR	polymerase chain reaction		
PDP	Personal Development Plan		
PDSA	plan, do, study, act		
PE	pulmonary embolism		
PEA	pulseless electrical activity		
PEFR	peak expiratory flow rate		
PG	postgraduate		
PICO	patient, intervention, comparison and outcome		
PICU	paediatric intensive care unit		

How to use your textbook

Features contained within your textbook

Each topic is presented in a double-page spread with clear, easy-to-follow diagrams supported by succinct explanatory text.

'Top tip' boxes give a summary of the topics covered in a chapter.

TOP TIPS

- Don't leave your SLEs and assessments to the last minute
- Every patient encounter can provide an opportunity for feedback
- Take time to reflect on your experiences and record this in your e-portfolio

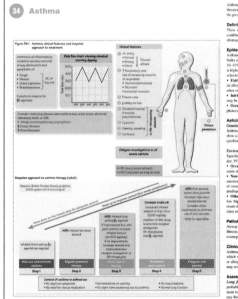

The anytime, anywhere textbook

Wiley E-Text

Your book is also available to purchase as a Wiley E-Text: Powered by VitalSource version – a digital, interactive version of this book which you own as soon as you download it.

Your Wiley E-Text allows you to:

Search: Save time by finding terms and topics instantly in your book, your notes, even your whole library (once you've downloaded more textbooks)

Note and highlight: Colour code, highlight and make digital notes right in the text so you can find them quickly and easily

Organize: Keep books, notes and class materials organized in folders inside the application

Share: Exchange notes and highlights with friends, classmates and study groups

Upgrade: Your textbook can be transferred when you need to change or upgrade computers

Link: Link directly from the page of your interactive textbook to all of the material contained on the companion website

The Wiley E-Text version will also allow you to copy and paste any photograph or illustration into assignments, presentations and your own notes.

To access your Wiley E-Text

- Visit   www.vitalsource.com/software/bookshelf/downloads   to download the Bookshelf application to your computer, laptop or mobile device.
- Open the Bookshelf application on your computer and register for an account.
- Follow the registration process.

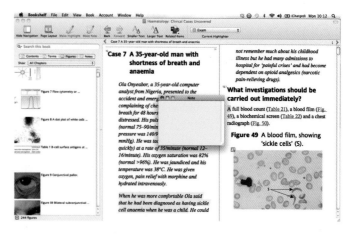

Wiley E-Text
Powered by VitalSource®

The VitalSource Bookshelf can now be used to view your Wiley E-Text on iOS, Android and Kindle Fire!

- **For iOS**: Visit the app store to download the VitalSource Bookshelf: http://bit.ly/17ib3XS
- **For Android**: Visit the Google Play Market to download the VitalSource Bookshelf: http://bit.ly/ZMEGvo
- **For Kindle Fire, Kindle Fire 2 or Kindle Fire HD**: Simply install the VitalSource Bookshelf onto your Fire (see how at http://bit.ly/11BVFn9). You can now sign in with the email address and password you used when you created your VitalSource Bookshelf Account.

   Full E-Text support for mobile devices is available at: http://support.vitalsource.com

CourseSmart

CourseSmart gives you instant access (via computer or mobile device) to this Wiley-Blackwell e-book and its extra electronic functionality, at 40% off the recommended retail print price. See all the benefits at: **www.coursesmart.com/students**

Instructors ... receive your own digital desk copies!

CourseSmart also offers instructors an immediate, efficient, and environmentally-friendly way to review this book for your course.

For more information visit www.coursesmart.com/instructors.

With CourseSmart, you can create lecture notes quickly with copy and paste, and share pages and notes with your students. Access your **CourseSmart** digital book from your computer or mobile device instantly for evaluation, class preparation, and as a teaching tool in the classroom.

Simply sign in at **http://instructors.coursesmart.com/bookshelf** to download your Bookshelf and get started. To request your desk copy, hit 'Request Online Copy' on your search results or book product page.

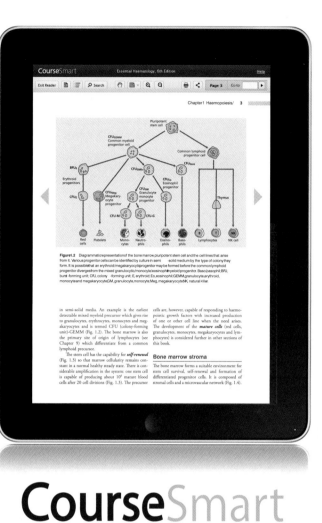

We hope you enjoy using your new book. Good luck with your studies!

Figure 1.1 Essential components of the F1 doctor's role

Essential list of clinical responsibilities

- Health and safety
- Critical incidents and how to report them
- Infection control
- Antibiotic prescribing
- ALS course
- Professionalism in the work place
- Blood transfusion competency assessment
- Effective hand over
- How to refer to psychiatry
- DVT prophylaxis
- Capacity and consent

Essential list of administrative jobs

- Find the F1 doctor that you are about to shadow
- Learn the layout of the hospital (e.g. where is the canteen?)
- Where do you get a bleep from?
- How do you access the computer?
- Is there a password?
- How does your e-portfolio work on the system?
- Which wards will you be covering?
- Is there a phlebotomist and what times do they work?
- Who is your educational supervisor?
- Meet the team
- Get your rota for your first job
- Ask about how to apply for holiday leave as there may be set periods when this is available
- When are you first on nights?
- Where is your accommodation, if available?
- The structure of the hospital and whom to contact re. problems or issues
- Equality and diversity training
- Death certification
- Domain accounts
- Clinical portal
- PACS system

Shadowing and induction

This chapter covers the new arrangements that are in place for the transition between medical student and foundation year 1 (F1) doctor.

The final year in medical school now places a far greater emphasis on learning in the workplace. You will therefore have undertaken:

- Clinical placements
- Student assistantships
- Shadowing
- Induction programme

Clinical placements

You will have typically undertaken these placements in primary, secondary or community healthcare settings and they are designed to ensure you have a broad experience of healthcare.

The key is to understand the working environment you are in and the care of the patient in that setting.

Student assistantships

This should have provided a number of hands-on learning experiences that allowed you to gain experience of working within clinical settings and to practice clinical jobs (Fig. 1.1). Most of your time would have been focused on the working role of the F1 doctor within that specialty.

Learning how to do your first F1 job
Shadowing

This is where you actually go to the site where you will be working as an F1 doctor and assist the F1 doctor whom you will replace following graduation in your first job. You should have already met the outcomes in the GMC's *Tomorrow's Doctors* (www.gmc-uk.org/education/undergraduate/tomorrows_doctors_2009.asp) by the time you start this attachment. You will have passed finals because the expected time of shadowing is the week before your job actually starts.

Induction

The induction period allows you to have a greater understanding of the working of the hospital and department in which you are now employed.

There is a great deal of overlap between shadowing and induction primarily because, in the past, students used to be only placed at their first job hospital on the day of starting the post. There then followed a period of lectures to introduce them to the hospital and the department in which they were to work.

Now it is expected that all students spend a period of time shadowing the F1 post that they are about to take up prior to their contract officially starting in August. The recommended length of the shadowing period should be a minimum of 4 days, and should be remunerated on a pro rata basic F1 salary.

So what do you need to do during the shadowing period to maximize the experience and ensure you are ready to take over the reins?

What you need to know

First you need to understand that the patients you are now seeing will be under your care. The outgoing F1 doctor will help you to get up to speed with the treatments and investigations for which they were admitted. If your team is on take then clerk as many of the patients yourself as you can because you will be looking after them. The shadowing period should where possible give you some out of hours experience. This can be very valuable, as your first experience of out of hours may not be with your own team but the hospital at night team.

Ask the outgoing F1 doctor how to make the most out of getting the work done in a timely fashion, which staff has the F1 found the most helpful, whom do they go to for help and advice, what time do lab results come back in the day, how do you get urgent investigations done? Time management will be key in reducing your understandable stress levels in the first few weeks (Fig. 1.1).

Who else should you meet?

The transition from student to professional doctor is not an easy one. You now have responsibility for the patients on your wards and working within your team. You will find it a lot busier than you imagined even after your clinical placements and assistantships.

Do not forget to look after yourself consider the following:

- Meet your educational supervisor as soon as you can
- Settle into your accommodation
- Get to know the staff and let them get to know you
- When in doubt ask
- Don't forget to eat
- The main focus is to get as much experience on the ward as possible, coupled with an understanding of how the hospital systems run

You will also get an opportunity to feed back on your shadowing experience so that this can be improved in subsequent years. Depending on where you have come from you may find some of the programme a repetition of the work you have done in your medical school. Remember, it is each hospital's responsibility to cover what they consider the essential elements they expect a new doctor to know. However, the real key to the shadowing period is the work you will do on the wards with the outgoing F1 doctor.

TOP TIPS

- If possible do the ALS course during the shadowing period
- Get a handover of patients from the current F1 doctor
- Ensure the list of patients is ready for your first day
- Make a list of jobs to be done when you start
- Get all forms filled in for the human resources department and complete the car permit forms before you start so you can focus on work from day one
- Unpack your bags so you can relax after the first few days at work
- Organize some after-work activities with your other F1s to get to know each other
- Meet as many of the ward staff as possible
- Find out where all the equipment is on the ward
- Find out what preparation you need to do for consultant ward round
- Find out the foibles of the firm
- Ask the F1 what procedures they got to grips with and where they felt they still had gaps

2 The e-portfolio – how to plan, manage and evidence your learning

Figure 2.1 A sample e-portfolio screenshot

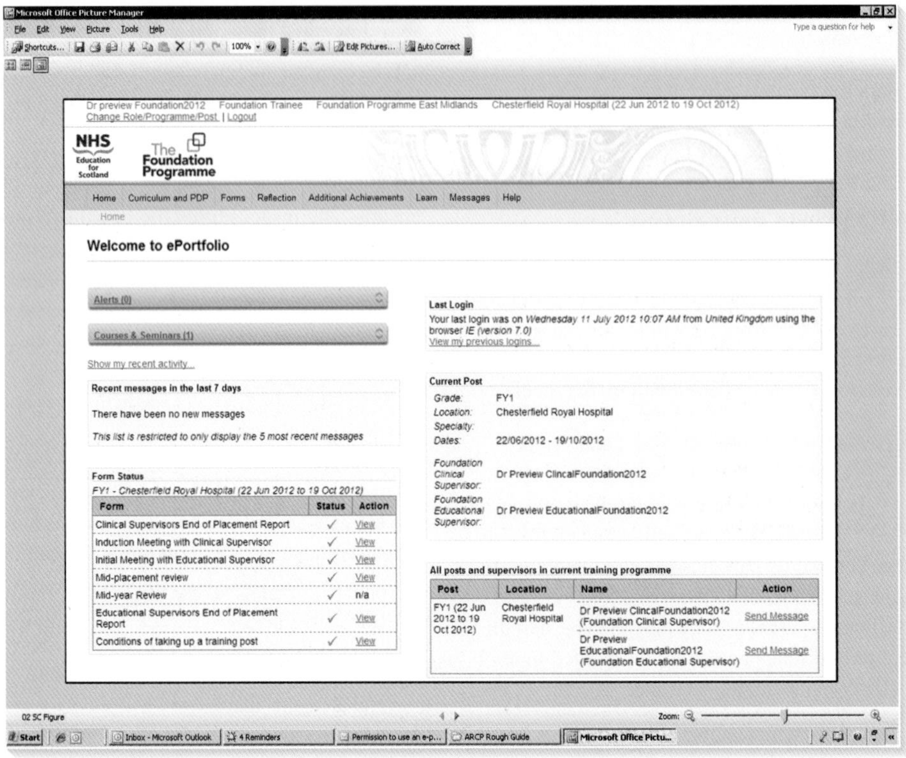

During the foundation programme (FP) you will be provided with access to an electronic portfolio (e-portfolio). Depending on which deanery/foundation school you attend, will determine which one (of the two) e-portfolio products will be used. A screenshot of the most commonly used e-portfolio is shown in Fig. 2.1. Both e-portfolios provide the same core content. This chapter covers how to make the most of your e-portfolio.

What is the e-portfolio for?

Your e-portfolio will be used to determine whether you have met the requirements for satisfactory completion of F1 and F2. You may also be invited to bring an abridged paper version of your portfolio to interviews for specialty training. Therefore it is essential that you plan your learning and gather evidence of your achievements throughout each foundation year.

The e-portfolio is designed to help you to:

- Plan and record your learning
- Record meetings with your educational and clinical supervisors
- Record supervised learning events and assessments
- Support reflective practice
- Capture additional evidence of achievements
- Provide evidence for sign-off at the end of F1 and F2

Who has access to my e-portfolio?

Your clinical supervisor, educational supervisor, foundation training programme director/tutor (FTPD/T), foundation school director (FSD) and manager (FSM), nominated e-portfolio administrators and a panel of Annual Review of Competence Progression (ARCP) members towards year-end have access to your e-portfolio. However, there are some sections which you can keep as private, e.g. your reflective learning reports.

What do I put in it?

Planning and recording your learning

The curriculum and personal development plan (PDP) section sets out the outcomes expected of a foundation doctor as described in the FP curriculum. It also includes space for you to identify additional outcomes.

It is important to remember that you are not expected to demonstrate all of the required curriculum outcomes at the beginning of the year but to develop them during your foundation programme.

When developing your own learning objectives using the PDP tool, make sure they are SMART:

Specific	Describe clearly what you intend to achieve and break this down into manageable chunks
Measurable	Consider what evidence you will present to demonstrate that you have met your learning objectives
Achievable	Set your learning objectives in partnership with your supervisor
Realistic	Explore what is feasible before setting your heart on any particular objective
Time-bound	When do you expect to achieve your specific, measurable, acceptable and realistic objective?

Recording your meetings with your clinical and educational supervisors

Meetings with your clinical supervisor You should meet with your clinical supervisor during the first week of each placement (induction meeting). You should discuss with your clinical supervisor what learning opportunities are available, what is expected of you and ensure you are familiar with the environment and location where you will be working. You should also discuss how to seek additional clinical support in and out of hours. This meeting must be recorded in the e-portfolio.

At the end of each placement, you should meet with your clinical supervisor to discuss the clinical supervisor's end of placement report. This report is an assessment based on your performance and builds on feedback from your colleagues/members of the Placement Supervision Group.

Meetings with your educational supervisor During your first meeting with your educational supervisor (initial meeting – within the first few weeks of F1/F2) you should agree your learning objectives. You will review these at subsequent educational supervisor meetings.

Before you meet with your educational supervisor for the first time, you should consider which of the curriculum outcomes you think you are likely to achieve in your first clinical placement and any others you would like to set (using the PDP tool). Many schools also provide detailed information about the sorts of learning opportunities available in each placement.

Similar to the meeting with your clinical supervisor, you are expected to meet with your educational supervisor at the beginning and near the end of each placement. This means that you should typically meet at least four times during the year.

Educational supervisor's meetings provide an opportunity for you to:
• Discuss and agree the educational supervisor's end of placement report
• Reflect on what went well in your last placement
• Reflect on areas you would like to focus on in your next placement
• Review your overall progress
• Agree when you will next review your learning objectives
• Discuss your career options

Supervised learning events and assessments

There are four supervised learning event (SLE) tools (see Chapter 3) which are designed to demonstrate engagement with the learning pro-

cess and enable constructive and immediate feedback on your performance in the workplace:
• Direct observation of procedural skills (DOPS)
• Mini clinical evaluation exercise (Mini-CEX)
• Case-based discussion (CBD)
• Developing the clinical teacher.
  In addition, there are five formal assessments tools:
• Team assessment of behaviour (TAB)
• Core procedures (F1)
• Clinical supervisor's end of placement reports
• Educational supervisor's end of placement reports
• Educational supervisor's end of year report.

Reflection

The ability to reflect on experiences and consider your learning needs and career aspirations is an important skill for all doctors. The reflection section includes a structured reflective log to help you reflect on your experiences as a foundation doctor, consider your learning needs and manage your career. See Chapter 4 for more details.

Additional evidence

In addition to demonstrating curricular outcomes, you can collect other evidence in your e-portfolio. The evidence gathered in this section could be particularly helpful when applying for specialty training and showing commitment to a clinical specialty. Examples of additional evidence include:
• Details of a quality improvement project (this is a requirement for satisfactory completion of F2)
• Course attendance
• Additional procedures
• Publications
• Exam certificates

Sign-off at the end of F1 and F2

All foundation doctors are subject to an ARCP review. The ARCP process is used to underpin and support F1/F2 sign-off. As part of this process, your e-portfolio will be scrutinized at the end of each foundation year.

An ARCP panel will make a judgement, based on the evidence you have provided (typically within the e-portfolio), against the requirements for satisfactory completion of each year. It is therefore vital that your e-portfolio accurately reflects your achievements and is managed effectively by you throughout the year.

Satisfactory completion of F1 will enable you to apply for full registration with the General Medical Council (GMC). Successful completion of F2 will result in the award of a foundation achievement of competence document (FACD), which allows you to start specialty training.

TOP TIPS

• Always be on the look out for learning opportunities
• Book appointments to see your clinical and educational supervisor(s) in advance
• Don't leave gathering e-portfolio evidence until the last minute!
• Put yourself in the role of an ARCP panellist; does your e-portfolio provide succinct evidence to show how you meet each of the requirements for F1/F2 sign off?

3 Supervised learning events and assessments

Figure 3.1   Supervised learning events (SLEs)

Tool	Frequency	Who should provide feedback?
Direct observation of doctor/patient interaction: • Mini-CEX • DOPS	3 or more mini-CEX per placement* Optional to supplement mini-CEX	• Named educational/clinical supervisor • Consultants and GP principals • Doctors more senior than F2 • Senior nurses (band 5 or above) • Allied health professionals
Case-based discussion (CBD)	2 or more per placement*	
Developing the clinical teacher	1 or more per year	

* Based on a clinical placement of 4-month duration

Figure 3.2   Assessments

Tool	Frequency	Who can assess?
Core procedures	Throughout F1	Assessors must be trained in assessment and feedback methodology. They must be able to competently perform the procedure themselves. This includes: • Consultants • GP principals • Specialist/specialty registrars • Staff grade/associate specialists • Doctors more senior than F1 • Fully qualified nurses • Allied healthcare professionals
Team assessment of behaviour (TAB)	At least once in F1 and F2. Your school will advise about timing	Assessors must include: • At least 2 doctors (including your designated clinical supervisor) but none may be other foundation doctors • At least 2 nurses (band 5 or above) • 2 or more allied health professionals (physiotherapists, occupational therapists, etc.) • At least 2 others (e.g. ward clerks, postgraduate programme administrators, secretaries, auxiliary staff)
Clinical supervisor's end of placement report	Once per placement*	Only the clinical supervisor should complete this report. The clinical supervisor should seek and record evidence from colleagues who form the Placement Supervision Group
Educational supervisor's end of placement report	Once per placement*	Only the educational supervisor can complete this report
Educational supervisor's end of year report	Once per year	Only the educational supervisor can complete this report

* Based on a clinical placement of 4-month duration

Regular feedback is central to foundation training. When coupled with personal reflection, constructive feedback will enable you to plan your learning and develop your knowledge, skills and competences. It can also be used to help identify any problems you are having early on, so that you and your supervisor can take steps to address these.

There are two structured approaches for constructive feedback during your foundation training:
• Supervised learning events (SLEs)
• Assessments
You should exploit every opportunity for feedback from colleagues and patients during your training.

This chapter covers SLEs and assessments. Giving feedback to medical students and other colleagues is covered in Chapter 18.

Supervised learning events (SLEs)

What are SLEs?

SLEs are tools for recording structured and immediate feedback from a more senior colleague. There are four tools that relate to different aspects of your practice as a foundation doctor (Fig. 3.1):
- **Direct observation of procedural skills (DOPS)**
- **Mini clinical evaluation exercise (Mini-CEX)**
- **Case-based discussion (CBD)**
- **Developing the clinical teacher**

When and how do you record a SLE?

You are expected to participate in SLEs throughout each placement and each foundation year. You are expected to complete a minimum number of each and are responsible for determining who provides feedback.

SLEs are accessed through your e-portfolio and require input and signature from both you and the person who facilitated the SLE/provided feedback. There are many ways the SLE forms can be completed (e.g. mobile access or sending your colleague an automated e-mail invitation known as a 'ticket'), however the key point is to record immediate and relevant feedback.

What is DOPS?

DOPS should be used to capture feedback on how you interact with a patient when undertaking a procedure. Each DOPS should be used for a different procedure and ideally should cover procedures other than the core procedures required for F1. It typically takes around 20 minutes to be observed undertaking each procedure and your colleague should allow an additional 5 minutes for immediate feedback.

What is mini-CEX?

Mini clinical evaluation exercise (Mini-CEX) supports feedback on a 'snapshot' of your clinical skills, e.g. how you undertake a mental state examination. The doctor/patient interaction typically takes around 20 minutes and immediate feedback around 5 minutes.

What is CBD?

CBD provides an opportunity for you to discuss clinical cases with a senior colleague. It is designed to support a structured discussion about your clinical reasoning. Examples of discussions as part of CBD include: safe prescribing and how you promote patient safety through good team working. It typically takes 20 minutes for each CBD including feedback and completion of the form.

What is developing the clinical teacher?

Developing the clinical teacher covers your teaching and/or presentation skills. This can be used for both one-to-one teaching and group teaching. The time needed to complete this SLE will depend on the teaching session topic and duration. Your colleague should allow sufficient time to provide feedback.

Assessments

How will you be assessed?

There are five forms of assessment (Fig. 3.2), which are all available in your e-portfolio:
- Team assessment of behaviour (TAB)
- Core procedural skills

- Clinical supervisor's end of placements reports
- Educational supervisor's end of placement reports
- Educational supervisor's end of year report

What is TAB?

TAB allows your colleagues to describe how you work as a member of the team, maintain trust, communicate verbally and how accessible you are. You need to select a range of 15 colleagues to provide multisource feedback on your performance, at least once during each year. Your educational supervisor will discuss the results with you. Before you can invite colleagues to contribute to a TAB round, you must complete a self-assessment (a self-TAB).

How are core procedural skills assessed?

During F1 you need to provide evidence that you can undertake all 15 core procedures listed in the curriculum, e.g. IV infusion of blood and blood products, injection of local anaesthetic to the skin, subcutaneous injection and performing and interpreting an ECG. The assessment is accessed through your e-portfolio by either sending your colleague a ticket or by entering the data yourself. The core procedures from F1 do not need to be repeated in F2, but evidence of the F1 sign-off is required for successful completion of the foundation programme. It should also be recognized that with practice, the foundation doctor is expected to demonstrate continuing improvement of skills in whichever procedure they perform.

What are the supervisor's reports?

At the end of each placement, your clinical supervisor will consult with colleagues (members of the Placement Supervision Group) to complete a structured report about your performance in the workplace. The report is mapped to the curriculum and is an important assessment.

Your educational supervisor will also complete end of placement and end of year reports/assessments. These reports will take account of your clinical supervisors' end of placement reports, your engagement with the training programme and any other assessments.

How to use feedback

In order to become more proficient as a doctor, you need to reflect on your experiences and in particular, the feedback you receive from colleagues. While it is great to receive positive feedback, constructive criticism about areas of relative weakness provides an opportunity for you to take steps to develop your skills. This opportunity should not be underestimated or overlooked.

Your educational supervisor will encourage you to reflect on how you feel in response to specific feedback, e.g. TAB and clinical supervisor's end of placement reports. This is an important step in helping to motivate you to identify your learning needs, any changes required and potential barriers. This process works best if there are specific examples for you to use/reflect on. Following any episode of reflection, you should consider developing an action plan using SMART objectives (see Chapter 2).

> **TOP TIPS**
>
> - Don't leave your SLEs and assessments to the last minute
> - Every patient encounter can provide an opportunity for feedback
> - Take time to reflect on your experiences and record this in your e-portfolio

4

Figure 4.1 An example of a reflective entry in a log

Date of critical incident: 18/12/10

Title: Inappropriate cardiac arrest call

Description – return to experience: A terminally ill patient had been admitted due to the carers inability to cope at that time. Therefore the patient was in hospital for social reasons. The arrest team had been called by a newly qualified nurse after the patient had been dizzy and collapsed. When the team arrived the patient was alert and certainly had not suffered a cardiac event. The patient was distressed by the presence of the team.

Education – making sense of situation: It was a surprise to be called to the arrest as the team had thought that that the patient was not for resuscitation. No DNAR had been completed and I should have ensured that this was discussed and in place. I was able to discuss with the team that no further action was needed at this time as the patient was now alert.

Analysis: I felt guilty that I had overlooked the resuscitation status of that patient but this on reflection was because we were not treating the patient for any current medical issues. I should have considered all aspects of the patient's care and not cut corners because there was nothing technically for me to do. I subsequently discussed the issue of resuscitation with the patient and he was clear that with his underlying condition he did not want to be considered for resuscitation. The notes were amended appropriately.

Action plan: I learnt that you need to consider all aspects of a patient's care from the time of their admission even if I have little to do with their subsequent care. I also learnt that we should have a standard review of patients' DNAR status with the team so all members know what is expected.

Time to complete: I took a couple of hours over this entry and did not write it all at once.

Private or shared: I have decided to share this with my educational supervisor so we could talk through how I felt and also what steps might be put in place with notes to reduce the possibility of this happening again.

This chapter covers the principles of reflection and describes why it is important that you develop your reflective skills for your professional development. It highlights a model for reflection to help you transform your clinical practice.

What is reflection?

Reflective learning is the process of being critical. This can mean thinking about a situation (and/or what is presented) and then deciding to accept or seek to change the situation. It can also involve accepting or seeking to change the information that has been presented.

Why is it important?

The skill of reflecting on your performance is vital in gaining a sense of how your practice can be improved. Reflection is not a natural ability and requires a systematic approach. It is not just the description of an experience but the analysis of this to improve your performance in patient care.

Using the e-portfolio to help your reflective practice

There is a reflective practice log within your e-portfolio. This provides a range of tools for you to record your own learning development. It is for you to decide if the reflective record is to remain private or whether you wish to share it with your educational supervisor. It forms part of your own continuous professional development which encompasses the following:

- Self-directed learning
- Professional self-awareness
- Learning developed in context
- Multidisciplinary and multilevel collaboration
- Your own learning needs and that of the organization
- An enquiry-based concept of professionalism

It is this type of critical thinking that underpins your future learning and educational needs but also places the patient as the central driver of your continued professional development.

A model for reflection

Your e-portfolio includes a structured reflection form to guide you through an incident or other clinical experience. While there are a range of possible structures and forms to guide your reflection, the key is to analyze what happened and consider changes in your behaviour or practice (Fig. 4.1).

Title of event
Description – return to experience
- What happened?
- Avoid waffle, be concise

Education – making sense of situation
- What influenced your action?
- How did you feel?
- Why did you feel this way?
- What were you trying to achieve?
- What was good about the experience and why?
- What was bad about the experience and why?
- What were the consequences for the patient, their family, yourself and colleagues?

Analysis
Examining components of the situation in detail coupled with critically analyzing the evidence is an essential stage in learning.
- What sense can be made of the situation?
- Assess your knowledge
- Evidence = provide relevant up-to-date information from literature or research
- Synthesis = integrate new knowledge with existing knowledge
- Identify and challenge assumptions and beliefs
- Explore alternatives: how would you do things differently in this situation? Or on reflection would you do the same again?
- If you were to do things differently, what might the consequences have been?

Action plan
This may result in a change of behaviour.
- If the situation arose again what would you do?
- Are there any preventative strategies that could be implemented?
- What do you need to learn?
- How will you go about gaining this new knowledge and/or skills?

Using this as the basis of your thinking will allow you to easily develop the requirements for the e-portfolio.

What examples can you use in your reflective log
Almost anything can be used as a means of reflecting and critically analyzing an event. It is perhaps best to start with one that is important and significant to you. Incidents are not just restricted to clinical events but may also include the following situations.

Procedural
- Lost X rays delay patient getting to theatre
- Missing notes
- Delay in discharge of patient while waiting for medication
- Missing or broken equipment on the ward preventing procedures being done
- No battery in bleep

Institutional (affecting patient care)
- Lack of locum cover out of hours
- No phlebotomy service at weekends
- No senior cover for junior doctors at night
- No formal hand over between shifts
- No hospital or departmental induction programme

It is worth emphasizing that good practice can also be used. Written ward-based protocols that everyone knows about and uses when a patient requires treatment is an example of good practice that may be lost on a more junior doctor if you do not reflect on why the procedure went well.

A reflective log will help you look more critically at the way you practice and improve the care you give to patients. It will be part of your continued professional development throughout your career and will form part of revalidation and relicensing.

Reflection should lead to an outcome either for you, the department or the institution.

TOP TIPS
- Choose a case that is important to you
- Be clear what the issue is for you and the patient
- Use positive examples as well as critical incidents
- Think what you could have done differently
- Have a positive action plan to move forward
- Record the information while it is still fresh in your mind
- Be sure to anonymize the data

Figure 5.1 The 4-stage career planning model

Career planning and decision-making has **four clear stages** and processes which are analogous to the patient care skills you are familiar with:

1. Self-assessment (taking a history)

- Exploring career values, motivators, preferences, personal strengths, limitations
- What do you define as rewarding work?
- What kinds of achievement are most important to you?
- What work–life factors do you wish to balance, now and in the future?
- What skills and interests do you have and want to optimize?
- Are there specific types of work and team environment you prefer?
- What are the practical factors such as finances, location, etc?

2. Career exploration (examination and investigations)

- Establishing options, alternatives and plan Bs, information gathering, networking, reality checking
- Attend career workshops in your foundation curriculum
- Reflect on your previous experiences, write career reflections, discuss career options, take a taster (or two)

Visit www.medicalcareers.nhs.uk
– a one-stop shop for all careers information

3. Decision-making (diagnosis)

Evaluating options, mapping skills and attributes against actual roles, considering options and preferences, clarifying personal factors, making choices

4. Plan implementation (treatment plan)

Detailed research into posts applied for, completing applications, updating your CV, preparing for assessments and interviews

Do not miss the first 2 stages; you would not jump straight to a diagnosis when dealing with your patients!

Based on Elton, Caroline and Reid, Joan (2010) The Roads to Success: A practical approach to career management for medical students, junior doctors (and their supervisors), 3rd edn. London: Postgraduate Deanery for Kent, Surrey and Sussex

This chapter covers:
- Career thinking and career planning skills
- Sources of career support
- Making career decisions

Medical careers offer a wide range of choices and are highly rewarding, but also require careful thought, planning and sometimes difficult choices. Opportunities to discuss and reflect on your career plans should occur at medical school and in the foundation programme. Sometimes you need help to find the right channel to deploy your valuable skills and talents. An interactive map will help you discover the many career options available to follow after medical school (http://careers.walesdeanery.org/map, last accessed 30 April 2013).

What should I aim for in my medical career?

Career choice, career development and career management are proactive lifelong processes which should be integral to every stage of medical education, training and work. For every individual, the 'perfect career' will look very different – it is unique to you.

Using the four-stage framework will help you to find support and information in an organized way (Fig. 5.1).

You may make several changes of direction within a career path and make lateral as well as vertical moves. This is almost inevitable as, over time, wider life priorities shift or the unexpected can happen.

Career discussions and where to find career support

Career discussions should form part of your appraisal with your educational supervisor. Other sources of impartial career support are available locally and in the deanery.

Tell them what your current goals are and which of the four stages you need help with as this will put someone in a better position to help you. You can seek help with career planning at any time from:
- Educational supervisors
- Foundation Programme Director/postgraduate (PG) centre manager/clinical tutor/Director of Medical Education
- Royal College tutor in every specialty in every hospital
- Speciality Training Programme Director and careers leader

If your career situation is complex, additional and impartial help may be needed. Any of the above can help you to arrange a confidential career meeting or remote discussion with one of your deanery careers team.

Be flexible: there are many great opportunities in medicine and a range of pathways to reach a long-term goal. Life contains mess and chance, which has an impact on all careers. View unplanned events as inevitable and as opportunities. This reality may be difficult to face and is made easier if you can develop the key career management skills of curiosity, persistence, flexibility, optimism and risk taking. You can become passionate about work as a result of participation – this is why the 'hidden' and shortage specialities are included in foundation programmes to let you explore options you may not have previously considered. No experience is ever a waste of time.

Exploring options in the foundation programme

Tasters: a taster is a period of time, usually 2–5 days, spent in a specialty the foundation doctor has not previously experienced, to develop insights into the work of a speciality and promote career reflection. Foundation programme directors can help arrange tasters. Guidance on tasters can be found on www.foundationprogramme.nhs.uk (last accessed 30 April 2013).

Learning career planning skills: you should take part in career development sessions as part of the generic curriculum. The opportunity to learn the skills to manage a medical career will be used throughout your working life.

Career reflection: a career reflection can be entered for each post on the e-portfolio. This provides a basis for career decision making as you explore your personal work values, practical skills and challenges and successes. Career reflections provide useful prompts when applying for specialty training, to demonstrate competencies and achievements, and provide evidence of how person specifications are met.

Be realistic: a career dream is great to have, but not a guarantee, and is attainable only in the context of your personal circumstances and the job market at any given time. Healthcare is continuously developing and services will look different in the future. An ageing population, changes in patient care pathways and new technology mean current employment opportunities may not exist in the future and more healthcare may be delivered in community and primary care environments.

Not everyone gets their first choice – what are you prepared to compromise on?

And never, ever be without a plan B!

Other career issues and changes to plan

Challenging periods within training or changes in personal circumstances prompt a need to reflect on a chosen career plan or to reset goals and options. Some individuals will choose or need to change direction.

Less than full time (LTFT), also called flexible, training: anyone who has well-founded reasons that prevent them from pursuing their career full-time is eligible, e.g.
- Being the parent of a young child/children
- Caring for an ill or disabled relative
- Having a disability or a health problem

Taking a break? There are many reasons for taking a career break and exploring other opportunities. All career breaks give valuable life experiences:
- Working overseas
- Travelling
- Time with family
- Time for further study
- Time for hobbies/business

Remember, there is no right or wrong career path – you are the best judge of which options meet your personal and professional needs.

TOP TIPS
- Start thinking about future career options early
- Explore widely and don't narrow your options too soon
- Keep an open mind
- Have a plan B and change career direction if plan A doesn't work out

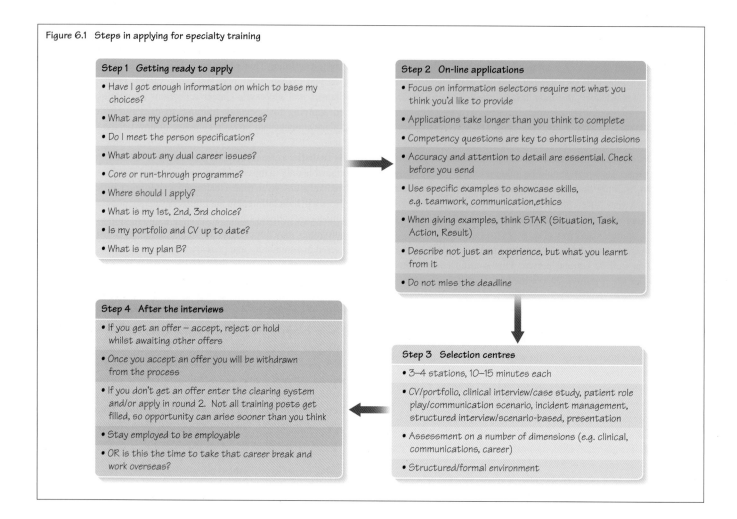

Figure 6.1 Steps in applying for specialty training

Step 1 Getting ready to apply

- Have I got enough information on which to base my choices?
- What are my options and preferences?
- Do I meet the person specification?
- What about any dual career issues?
- Core or run-through programme?
- Where should I apply?
- What is my 1st, 2nd, 3rd choice?
- Is my portfolio and CV up to date?
- What is my plan B?

Step 2 On-line applications

- Focus on information selectors require not what you think you'd like to provide
- Applications take longer than you think to complete
- Competency questions are key to shortlisting decisions
- Accuracy and attention to detail are essential. Check before you send
- Use specific examples to showcase skills, e.g. teamwork, communication,ethics
- When giving examples, think STAR (Situation, Task, Action, Result)
- Describe not just an experience, but what you learnt from it
- Do not miss the deadline

Step 4 After the interviews

- If you get an offer – accept, reject or hold whilst awaiting other offers
- Once you accept an offer you will be withdrawn from the process
- If you don't get an offer enter the clearing system and/or apply in round 2. Not all training posts get filled, so opportunity can arise sooner than you think
- Stay employed to be employable
- OR is this the time to take that career break and work overseas?

Step 3 Selection centres

- 3–4 stations, 10–15 minutes each
- CV/portfolio, clinical interview/case study, patient role play/communication scenario, incident management, structured interview/scenario-based, presentation
- Assessment on a number of dimensions (e.g. clinical, communications, career)
- Structured/formal environment

This chapter covers:
- Steps to follow when making career decisions
- A description of processes – application and selection
- Myths about speciality training

Career paths into and through specialty training require research and planning. Research beforehand enables you to plan your application well in advance.

Exploration of the options

Information on person specifications, vacancies, competition ratios, entry requirements and application procedures are widely available. Whilst more information is always useful, this may have little impact on final decision making when geography and social networks are deemed more important than speciality opportunities as career decision drivers – see Step 1 (Fig. 6.1).

- www.medicalcareers.nhs.uk (last accessed 30 April 2013) – the largest and most comprehensive UK medical careers website, with information on all the specialties, case studies, review of the wider options and links to all other sites.

- www.mmc.nhs.uk (last accessed 30 April 2013) – medical specialty training website with details of application processes, person specifications, eligibility criteria, competition ratios and tips on preparing for the interview.

- Deaneries, Royal College websites and NHS Jobs website have details of vacancies.

You can discuss your options with your educational supervisor, foundation programme director, the Director of Medical Education and the deanery careers team.

Career decisions will be influenced by personal circumstances and may change over time as life events occur and personal experience influences choices. Approximately 10–15% of all doctors change specialty at some point in their careers.

Career structure of your chosen specialties

Specialty training programmes are organized in various ways and it is important to be clear about the pathway before you apply.

Run through

Some specialties operate run through training programmes and progression is automatic subject to satisfactory progress and achievement of competences: paediatrics, obstetrics and gynaecology, general practice, public health, clinical radiology, histopathology, ophthalmology, clinical pathology, medical microbiology, clinical neurosurgery and academic clinical fellowship.

Uncoupled

Other specialties are split into 'core' and 'higher' training. These uncoupled specialties give 2 or 3 years of core training after which a further application for higher training is required – medicine, surgery, psychiatry, anaesthetics and emergency medicine.

Make sure you check the rules for each time you make an application.

Application process timelines

The main annual recruitment round 1 opens before Christmas for posts starting the following August. Round 2 follows to fill posts not appointed in round 1. Adverts on the NHS Jobs website (and in the BMJ) are followed by an on-line application process (see Step 2 in Fig. 6.1). Note deadlines and give yourself enough time to submit your application.

Application portals are managed by Royal Colleges and postgraduate deaneries – this varies between specialties.

You will be asked for the names of two referees – make sure you have asked them.

For GP programmes application is followed by sitting a machine marked test – note the date.

Candidates for speciality training are asked to indicate their preferred location/deanery of training programme.

If shortlisted you are invited to attend a selection centre – the invitation will outline the methodology of selection (see Step 3). If you have a registered disability you may wish to declare this on your application so that adjustments can be made at the selection centre.

Interview/selection process

First impressions count. In the first 5 minutes of an interview you will convey information by:body language (55%), tone and pace of your voice (38%) and the words you say (7%). It always helps to practice your interview skills.

There are four basic underlying questions for interviewees to answer:
- Why have you applied for this job/speciality?
- What can you do for us? (What skills, knowledge and intellectual ability can you offer?)
- What kind of person are you? (What are your attitudes, values, motivation levels? Do you have the ability to get on with others, work in a team?)
- What distinguishes you from all the other applicants?

Applicant etiquette

- If you decide not to attend or to withdraw from an interview notify the recruiters
- Be on standby – you may receive an interview invitation at short notice
- Arrive with all requested documents and your portfolio
- Schedules on the day can be unpredictable, so arrive in plenty of time
- Do not accept a post which you don't intend to take up (see Step 4)
- Understand the rules about holding offers and acceptance or rejection of offers

Less than full time (LTFT) training

LTFT training is possible in all speciality training programmes. There is often a question on the application form asking if you wish to train LTFT. If you tick 'yes' this answer remains confidential until after the selection process, i.e. those scoring your application and assessing you at the selection centre are not aware that you have requested LTFT training.

Myths about speciality training applications

- You only get one chance a year to apply for specialty training
- Working in a fixed term specialty post will count against me in the future
- Once in a specialty it is well nigh impossible to change
- Applications to change specialty will be unfavourably viewed
- If I apply to more than one specialty the others will find out
- If a consultant expresses a view on a career route it is the absolute truth

None of the above is correct!

Entry into speciality training is not the only route after foundation; you may decide to gain further general or overseas experience before specializing.

You are the sole owner of your career, and your willingness to research options, ask questions, reflect on experiences and show commitment during application processes will help to determine your long-term success.

> **TOP TIPS**
>
> - Prepare well
> - Follow instructions and meet deadlines
> - Don't apply for a job you won't accept.

Figure 7.1 Key relationships for quality improvement

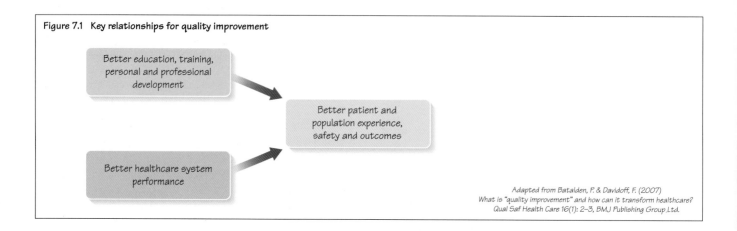

Better education, training, personal and professional development

Better healthcare system performance

Better patient and population experience, safety and outcomes

Adapted from Batalden, P. & Davidoff, F. (2007)
What is "quality improvement" and how can it transform healthcare?
Qual Saf Health Care 16(1): 2–3, BMJ Publishing Group.Ltd.

This chapter covers the principles of quality improvement and clinical leadership. All members of the healthcare team share a common goal – to improve the health of patients and the public.

As a foundation doctor, you have a critical role to play in contributing to the continuous improvement of care to improve patient outcomes, safety and experience. This includes following national or local guidelines and protocols, participating in surveys, and leading or contributing to quality improvement projects (see Chapter 8).

What is quality improvement?

'Quality improvement' describes the efforts of all members of the healthcare team to transform healthcare for the benefit of patients. When considering the healthcare team, you should include patients and their carers.

Since the mid-1990s the NHS has used the term 'clinical governance' to describe its approach to maintaining and improving the quality of care. Sir Liam Donaldson, who was the Chief Medical Officer for England, defined clinical governance as:

> A framework through which NHS organisations are accountable for continually improving the quality of their services and safeguarding high standards of care by creating an environment in which excellence in clinical care will flourish.

Improving healthcare for the benefit of patients

The model shown in Fig. 7.1 identifies two inter-related vehicles for improving patient outcomes:
- Changes to how the healthcare system operates (process of care)
- Changes to the capabilities of staff, i.e. through the education, training and continued personal and professional development of the healthcare team

You should consider four questions when considering how you might improve the operation of the healthcare system or enhancing the skills of the team:

1 What is the context?
- Before you consider the evidence from other settings, it is important to understand how and why care is delivered in a particular way in your organization
- You should talk to colleagues and ask for copies of any papers that explain the rationale for a particular approach. This will help you identify particular barriers to change and help you narrow the search when looking for evidence of what has worked in similar situations
- You should also engage patients, carers and colleagues when exploring the opportunities to improve care. Feedback from patients and their carers is particularly influential when making a case for change with management colleagues
- You should not be afraid to question the status quo

2 What has worked in similar situations?
- You will need to apply an evidence-based approach to the identification and critical appraisal of the research evidence. This includes considering whether it is applicable to your environment

3 How will you evaluate the impact of any change?
- Chapter 8 covers two approaches to measuring change: 'Plan, do, study, act' and 'Audit'
- You should always try and keep your project simple and gather readily available and meaningful data

4 How will you lead and implement changes?
- This is your opportunity to develop and demonstrate your leadership skills. In particular, you should develop a project proposal and enlist the support of other to introduce the changes

Leading and implementing changes

Leadership is not just about status and titles. It is about taking responsibility for ensuring that your patients benefit from the best possible care. All leaders in the health service share a common goal – to continuously improve patient safety, outcomes and experience.

As a member of a team, you will need to recognize and negotiate with your colleagues when you should follow and when you should lead. As an F1 doctor you will take a lead role in supporting medical students during their student assistantships. In F2, you will supervise F1 doctors, lead the resuscitation of patients, direct ward rounds and organize handovers. By the end of your foundation training, you must also provide evidence that you can lead a quality improvement project, e.g. a 'plan, do, study, act' or audit (see Chapter 8).

Some of the core skills of a leader include:
- Articulating a vision
- Developing and describing a plan to realize the vision
- Inspiring others to follow

However, you can also show leadership by encouraging improvement and innovation. This includes questioning the status quo and encouraging dialogue and debate with your colleagues. Making a difference to patients and the public should be the key to these discussions.

TOP TIPS

- Question the status quo
- Use the tools on the e-portfolio to reflect on your leadership style and develop your skills
- Keep evidence that you have completed the National Trainee Survey, and any other surveys or activities designed to improve the quality of your education and training
- Plan your quality improvement project early

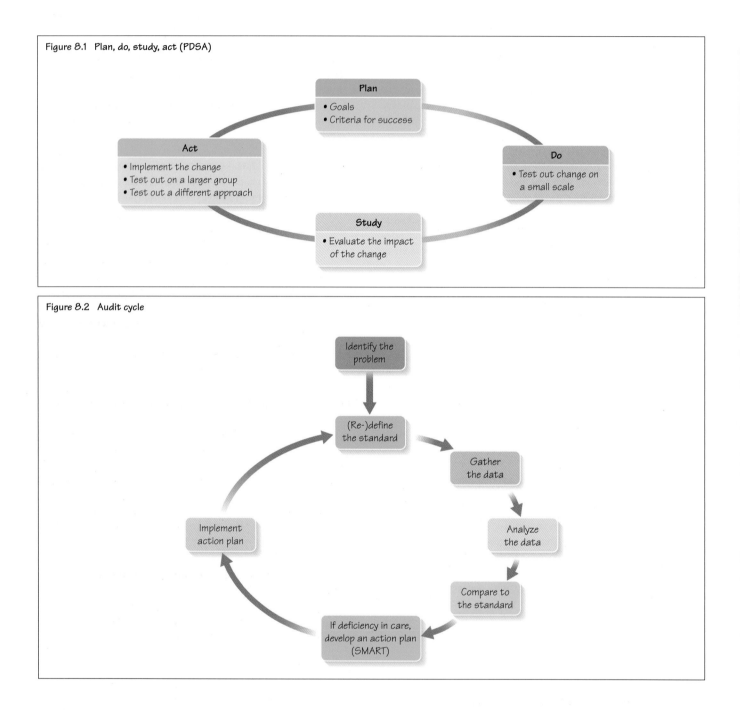

Figure 8.1 Plan, do, study, act (PDSA)

Plan
- Goals
- Criteria for success

Do
- Test out change on a small scale

Study
- Evaluate the impact of the change

Act
- Implement the change
- Test out on a larger group
- Test out a different approach

Figure 8.2 Audit cycle

- Identify the problem
- (Re-)define the standard
- Gather the data
- Analyze the data
- Compare to the standard
- If deficiency in care, develop an action plan (SMART)
- Implement action plan

This chapter covers two common approaches to assess, evaluate and improve patient care: plan, do, study, act (PDSA) and audit. As part of your foundation training, you must provide evidence that you have managed, analyzed and presented at least one quality improvement project. If you plan your project early, you can also use it to demonstrate commitment to your preferred specialty when applying for the next stage of your training.

Plan, do, study, act (PDSA)

PDSA is a tool to deliver and test improvements in patient care. The key to PDSA is to start small, trial the proposed change using repeated cycles and use the data to plan larger scale improvements.

If you engage your colleagues in the process, you are more likely to successfully roll-out any changes. For example, you and your colleagues could use PDSA cycles to:

- Test out a new process for prioritizing referrals
- Gather feedback from patients
- Reduce the risk of prescribing errors
  There are four stages (Fig. 8.1).

Plan
- There are two questions underpinning any changes:
  ○ What are you trying to achieve?
  ○ How will you know if the change is an improvement?
- In setting goals, you should align them to any national goals and ensure that they have clear and measurable targets

Do
- You should trial the change on a small scale, e.g. with patients attending a clinic on a single afternoon
- It is best to trial the change with colleagues who are committed to the project

Study
- As part of the planning stage, you should have identified key outcome measures, e.g. number of patients seen, waiting time and proportion of patients providing feedback
- When evaluating the impact of the change, you can compare data before and after
- You and your colleagues will learn from changes that work and don't work

Act
- At this stage, there are three options:
  ○ Develop another strategy
  ○ Plan a larger scale study
  ○ Plan full implementation
- You should only make changes to clinical practice when you're confident you have considered and tested all the possible ways of making an improvement

Audit
Audit measures current practice against a defined standard. It asks the question: Are we actually doing what we should be doing? However, audit is not just about quantifying a deficiency in patient care – it should be used to identify and test possible solutions.

There are five stages to the audit cycle (Fig. 8.2).

Stage 1 – what problem would you like to fix?
- Audit projects tend to be most effective when the entire team is committed to fixing a specific problem, e.g. prescription errors. You should try and find something you are interested in
- Your local quality improvement or audit lead may be able to help identify a topic and provide training and support

Stage 2 – what are you seeking to achieve?
- This is about the defining the standard.
- The standard should be derived from clinical practice guidelines or the medical literature. For example, the National Institute for Health

and Care Excellence (NICE) depression guideline states that, 'People with depression that has not responded to initial treatment within 6 to 8 weeks should have their treatment plan reviewed'
- It can often be challenging determining what level should be applied. There are three options to setting the level of the standard:
  ○ Minimum standard – the lowest acceptable standard of performance. The minimum standard distinguishes between acceptable and unacceptable practice
  ○ Ideal standard – the best possible standard of performance. This describes the standard of care you would expect under ideal conditions, with no constraints
  ○ Optimum standard – this lies between the minimum and the ideal. This describes the standard of care most likely to be achieved under normal conditions of practice
- To make the standard clinically useful, you should describe it as a percentage. e.g. '98% of people with depression that has not responded to initial treatment should have a copy of their treatment plan review documented in their notes'

Stage 3 – how are you going to gather and analyze the data?
- You should try and keep this as simple as possible and where possible draw upon computerized records. If you are reviewing case notes, make sure that you do not make it difficult for your colleagues to access them when needed
- Data analysis includes comparing what you found with the agreed standard. Where possible, you should try and clarify why the standard was not met, e.g. incomplete case notes, clinician forgot to review the treatment plan or patient did not attend appointment

Stage 4 – what changes or improvements need to be made?
- One of the most effective ways of developing an action plan that is likely to work, is to discuss the results with your colleagues
- You and your colleagues, should develop an action plan that sets out what needs to be done, how it will be done, who is going to do it and by when
- For example, you could develop stickers for patient case notes reminding clinicians that they need to review the treatment plan at 8 weeks if the patient has not responded to treatment

Stage 5 – how will you demonstrate that you have made a difference?
- After you have implemented the action plan, you should repeat the audit cycle to determine whether the actions have been effective, or whether further improvements are needed

---

TOP TIPS
- Plan your quality improvement project early
- Select a topic that interests you and/or relates to your preferred career choice
- Submit your results for a poster presentation or for publication

Figure 9.1 Examples of bad news

- Telling a patient their operation is postponed/cancelled
- That you need to repeat an investigation that they found 'uncomfortable'
- That they cannot yet go home
- That they need an operation
- That they will be on long-term medication/treatment
- That they have to stop or curtail a favourite pastime
- That their illness is hereditary
- That there is no further treatment for them
- That they have cancer
- That they are terminally ill

Figure 9.2 Handling complaints

- Get the facts as viewed by the patient or relative
- Try to do this in a calm environment
- Take the person to a private area or room
- You may well need a witness to help you record or verify what was said
- Decide whom is the most appropriate person to deal with the situation
- Explain what you are going to do and whom you might need to refer to
- Give the patient or relative a timeframe for when you will get back to them
- Document the complaint in the notes
- Speak to your supervisor
- Stay calm

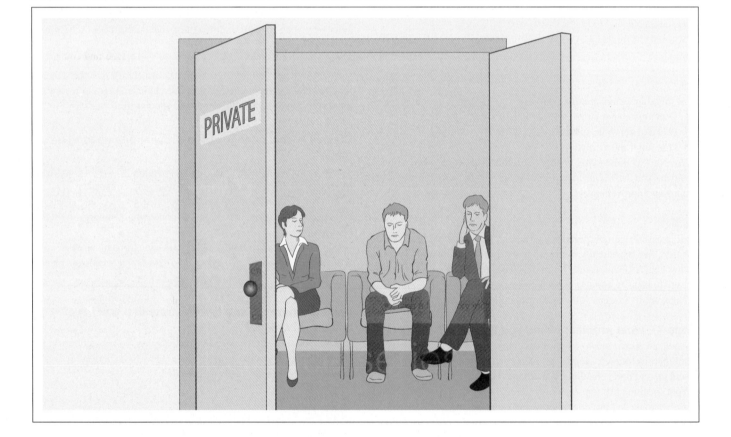

This chapter covers two of the most difficult and stressful tasks you will have to undertake as a doctor – breaking bad news and handling complaints. These issues will have a major impact not only on the lives and health of your patients but also on the way that you approach your professional life. Breaking bad news will become a common part of your professional career and it is essential that you understand the best way to approach the event. Hopefully handling complaints will be an in frequent part of your career but again it is essential to understand the best ways to approach these problems to minimize the risk of escalation and ending up in court.

Breaking bad news

It is unlikely as a student that you will have been the main person to break bad news to a patient or a relative. It is, however, much more likely that you will be in a position to have to discuss difficult issues with patients. Bad news covers an array of situations.

While some of the scenarios (Fig. 9.1) are clearly 'bad news' it is the patient's own reaction to what you say that really defines the situation. A cancelled appointment may mean very little to you but can have a dramatic effect on the patient and their family. It can cause all sorts of problems with their work and increase their anxiety and stress levels. Other patients may be relieved to hear that they have a serious illness after months of not knowing and repeated investigations. Your handling of the situation, which may not be unique to you but certainly is to the patient, will set the ongoing tone for your relationship with this individual and their family.

As a foundation doctor it is very likely that more senior members of the team will undertake the role of breaking more serious medical bad news to a patient and their relatives. It is essential that you learn as much as you can from your seniors as you will be the one to do this in the future. These situations can provide excellent cases for your reflective log in your e-portfolio and the ongoing development of your skills.

Ask to join the doctor or nurse who is giving bad news and consider the following:
• Who else is in the room?
• Where did the doctor or other member of the team decide to give the news?
• Were you interrupted or likely to be?
• How much time was given to the patient?
• Did the patient ask questions?
• Did they look as if they understood the issues?
• What follow up was offered to ensure the messages had got across?
• What would you have done differently?

There are some common approaches that can help when breaking bad news:
• Know your facts
• Ensure you have time to spend with the patient
• Check their understanding of what you have said
• Ensure you or another member of staff follow up the session to further support the patient
• Ensure you are not interrupted
• Use a private side room if possible
• Don't use jargon
• Empathize with the patient

Breaking bad news can be traumatic for you as well so ensure that you have someone to talk through how the episode went and reflect on how it might be improved. Your educational supervisor would be an appropriate person to discuss this with and could form part of one of your meetings in reviewing the content of your e-portfolio. This will help improve your skills in this area to the benefit of patient care.

Handling complaints

This is a stressful event but again one that is likely to happen to every doctor at some time in their career. Complaints are not always related to medical error but run the entire gamut of experiences related to patient care:
• Cancelled operations
• Postponed outpatient appointments
• Delayed investigations

• Lack of beds
• Poor food
• No one to feed the patient
• Delayed admission/discharge
• Rude staff
• Lack of information

It is again unlikely that you will have had much experience in dealing with patient complaints as an undergraduate but patients may well use you as the first point of contact because you are on the wards and accessible to them. No complaints are trivial and should all be dealt with by the appropriate individuals who can help facilitate a swift resolution (Fig. 9.2).

Your hospital will also have a policy on handling complaints and you should have been made aware of this during shadowing and induction. You certainly need to be aware of and make reference to this policy in any dealing you have with regard to patient complaints.

In more serious cases anyone involved with the case may be asked to provide written evidence on the incident and give oral evidence to an internal panel. This is where you will be pleased that the patient's file has excellent and comprehensive entries.

If you are asked to present evidence then consider the following:
• Consult the notes, particularly your entries
• Stick to the facts of the case exactly and only what you have been asked
• Do not use emotive language in your response
• Have your educational supervisor review the tone and content of what you have written
• Ring your medical defence union for advice
• Take a colleague with you if you have to present oral evidence
• Reflect on the lessons that can be learnt from the experience
• Have a debrief with your educational supervisor

While you may not be the focus of the complaint it is still a stressful experience to give written or oral evidence. It is also likely to be your first experience of this situation, which can add to your stress. You need to ensure you have the proper support from your educational supervisor and it also can be useful to have peer support if you have to give evidence. This helps when reflecting on how the process worked as getting another person's perspective often reveals that you have answered the questions well.

Breaking bad news and handling complaints need a whole-team approach and support from your supervisors and peers. These are not situations that should be approached alone but require knowledge of the trust processes, empathy and understanding. Stepping back from the emotion of the situation and reflecting and giving yourself time to think is a skill that needs to be developed to help you cope with these difficult situations.

TOP TIPS
• Stay calm
• Document everything
• Use a private room to talk
• Follow up with another meeting
• Use written material to give to the patient
• Involve your team
• Don't promise anything you can't deliver

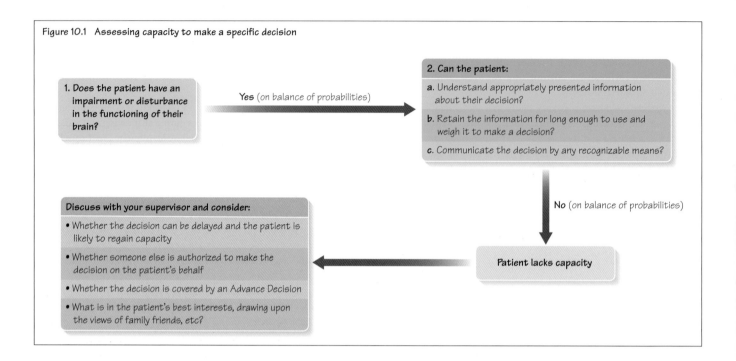

Figure 10.1 Assessing capacity to make a specific decision

1. Does the patient have an impairment or disturbance in the functioning of their brain?

Yes (on balance of probabilities)

2. Can the patient:

a. Understand appropriately presented information about their decision?

b. Retain the information for long enough to use and weigh it to make a decision?

c. Communicate the decision by any recognizable means?

No (on balance of probabilities)

Patient lacks capacity

Discuss with your supervisor and consider:

• Whether the decision can be delayed and the patient is likely to regain capacity

• Whether someone else is authorized to make the decision on the patient's behalf

• Whether the decision is covered by an Advance Decision

• What is in the patient's best interests, drawing upon the views of family friends, etc?

Caring for patients who refuse treatment is one of the greatest challenges as a foundation doctor. Although, there is a presumption of capacity, you may fear that the patient's judgement is compromised and failure to act could prolong suffering or risk death. It is equally important to ensure that patients who agree to treatment have capacity.

This chapter covers the assessment of capacity and provides guidance about what you should do if your patient lacks capacity to make a specific decision.

What is mental capacity?

Mental capacity is decision-specific and time-specific. It is the ability to understand the proposed options and retain the information for long enough to consider the risks and benefits and make an informed decision.

Therefore every time you are considering an investigation or treatment, you should ask yourself the question, 'Can the person make this decision at this time?'

Principles

There are three guiding principles:
• Presume that the patient has capacity unless there is evidence to the contrary
• People who have capacity may make unwise or eccentric decisions
• Do all you can to maximize a person's capacity

Supporting patients to make decisions

Being a patient can be scary. Of its nature, the doctor/patient relationship is asymmetrical and the decisions under consideration are life changing. It is important to make sure that your patient is given time and space to consider their options and make an informed decision.

Mental illness, delirium, dementia, stroke and many other conditions can impair brain functioning and render the patient unable to make decisions. However, the impact of these conditions can fluctuate over time. Patients may be able to make simple decisions but struggle with more complex ones.

There are a number of strategies that should be considered to maximize the patient's capacity to make a decision:
• Don't rush decisions – allow your patient sufficient time to make decisions
• Provide written or audio information about the options
• Discuss decisions in a place and time when the patient is likely to be able to retain the information, e.g. in a private room
• Ask if the patient would like to bring or involve a friend, relative or an advocate
• Plan for foreseeable changes in the patient's capacity to make decisions

You should seek advice from other colleagues (e.g. your supervisor, nursing colleagues, liaison psychiatry) about the best possible strategy.

Two-stage test of mental capacity

When assessing capacity there are two stages to the test and the standard is based on the balance of probabilities (Fig. 10.1).
1 Does the person have an impairment of mind or is there some sort of disturbance affecting the way their mind or brain works either on a temporary or a permanent basis (diagnostic test)?
2 If so, does that impairment or disturbance mean that the person is unable to make the decision in question at the time that it needs to be made (functional test)?

Stage 1 – diagnostic test

When considering whether a patient lacks capacity, you must first consider whether there is an underlying condition causing the disturbance. There are numerous conditions that could impair or disturb the way in which the mind or brain works. The more common conditions include:
• Delirium
• Dementia
• Substance use
• Mental health disorder
• Stroke or brain injury
• Learning disability

Stage 2 – functional test

The functional test of capacity comprises four components: understanding, retention, use and weighing up, and communication. You must ensure that you have presented the risks and benefits of the options in a way that the patient can understand. You could ask the patient to explain the options in their own words. This will enable you to assess whether the patient has understood and can retain the information.

When the patient makes a decision, you should ask for an explanation of their reasoning to confirm that they have used the information in their deliberations. The patient can communicate the decision by any recognizable means, e.g. in writing, using a communication board or voice synthesizer.

Acting in the patient's best interests

If on the balance of probabilities, you believe that the patient lacks capacity to make the decision, you should record your assessment in the notes and involve your supervisor in determining what further action should be taken. It may be the case that the decision can be postponed, especially if there is a chance that the patient's condition is likely to fluctuate or improve.

The patient may have appointed a substitute decision maker (e.g. someone with lasting power of attorney) or issued an Advance Decision to direct treatment. The guiding principle is acting in the patient's best interests and respecting their wishes.

> **TOP TIPS**
> • Do all you can to help improve the patient capacity to make a decision
> • Remember to fully document your assessment of capacity

11 Handover and communicating with colleagues

Figure 11.1 Out of hours handover form

St Elsewhere and Somewhere Hospitals
Out of Hours Handover

Handed over by ....Dr A.......

Handing over to ....Dr B.......

Day covered by this handover (Please circle): Mon (Tue) Wed Thu Fri Sat Sun

Patient surname, Forename, Date of Birth, NHS/Hospital no.	Responsible consultant, Patient current location	Diagnosis/Problem list Differential diagnosis (include any risks or warnings)	Reason for handover	Outstanding issues (tasks to be done)	Aims and limitations of treatment (e.g. Resus/ITU/Ventilation/ Inotropes/Active/Palliative/ Surgery – Y/N)
SMITH A 18/4/48 T24763	DR MANN WARD 4	ABDO PAIN ? UTI ? CONSTIPATION	ON GOING INVESTIGATIONS ? I.V. ANTIBODIES	BLOODS ULTRASOUND	CHECK RESULTS POTENTIAL DISCHARGE Discharge over w/e (Y) N
JONES T 7/9/50 T47523	DR MANN WARD 4	R. UPPER QUADRANT PAIN ? GALL STONES ? ULCER	W/S NEEDS BOOKING + ENDOSCOPY	W/S ENDOSCOPY	PAIN RELIEF + FLUIDS Discharge over w/e Y (N)
SEGUR P 3/9/58 T43222	DR DEAN WARD 8	CHEST PAIN ? MI ? PE	BLOODS CXR REFERRAL TO CARDIOLOGIST	CXR ? CTPA	MOVE TO CCU REPORT ECG Discharge over w/e Y (N)
ROBERTS D 10/10/39 T32478	DR DEAN WARD 9	OFF FEET CONFUSED ? STROKE	TRANSFER WARD NEURO OPINION PHYSIOTHERAPY	BLOODS CT SCAN CXR	PALLIATIVE CARE DISCUSS WITH RELATIVES Discharge over w/e Y (N)
TROON S 23/4/53 T63247	DR MANN WARD 2	CHEST INFECTION ? PNEUMONIA	REFER PHYSIO	CXR BLOODS I.V. ANTIBIOTICS	VENTILATION IF REQUIRED Discharge over w/e (Y) N

Signature ....D. Gallen.......

The job of being a doctor involves communicating and ensuring that whatever is said or written down is accurately translated by anyone who hears or reads the message to ensure the safety of patients. This chapter covers how best to communicate with colleagues and the role of leadership in communication

Effective communication with colleagues

Communicating with colleagues is clearly not just restricted to the handover period but includes all interactions with all members of the team. To communicate effectively with your colleagues to improve patient care, you must:

• Display understanding of your personal role within the team and be able to support the team leader

• Listen to the views of other healthcare professionals

• Take leadership roles and delegate appropriately in the context of your own competence

• Meticulously cross check instructions and actions with your colleagues

• Be able to identify and deal with poor performance in yourself and in others

So communication is more than just what you say or write but involves a real understanding of the roles and responsibilities of all team members.

• Do you know how much help and support the nursing staff can give you?

• Do you know what specialized roles some of them have?

• Do you know how to make a referral to and access the allied health professionals linked to your ward and specialty?

Spending time finding out these facts will help you function better in the team and ensure that patients have access to the right help and support. These are also the staff members who will be filling in your TAB forms so they will be commenting on your performance!

Safe handover

One of the most important tasks for patient safety is robust handover and clear communication with your fellow doctors and other members of the healthcare team. Handover normally takes place at the beginning and end of each day, but because of the changing shift patterns due to the working time directive it can, and often does, occur outside the normal times. This makes it even more important to get this right as handover in the middle of the night may not have the same formality as those done first thing in the morning.

Whatever the time you should have a clear action plan as to what and whom you are handing over or taking on responsibility for. You need to be able to prioritize both the work and the urgency of the medical conditions of your patients.

Consider the following:
- Which patients are the sickest?
- Which patients need reviewing?
- What investigations have been done and what results are awaited?
- What further tests need to be done?
- What further jobs remain, e.g. drug forms, blood tests for next day?
- Do you need to speak to any relatives or carers?

Don't forget this is a team handover and it is not just about the doctors. Make sure you have written down everything you need from the handover and that you have equally kept good notes to pass on at the end of your shift. Also be clear whom you are working with and where you can get help.

Many hospitals now have a standard template for handover and this can reduce errors and ensure the whole team understand the work to be done (Fig. 11.1). You should meticulously cross check instructions and actions with your colleagues.

Leadership and communication

The ability to understand the role of leaders is an essential competency for any doctor. While it is right to emphasise the need for good team work it is also essential to have good leaders who can communicate and express what the team needs to focus on. Leadership includes being able to recognize and take steps to address underperformance in an individual or the team.

Dealing with poor performance in others

This may be your first job and it can be difficult to understand the reasons for poor performance in other members of the team. You have a duty to ensure that patients receive the best possible care and recognize that problems within the team can have a negative effect on care.

It is always worth reflecting whether the problem in the team is due to your own approach before looking to others. Stress can play a large part in the way you or members of the team react to situations and can manifest itself in many ways:
- Avoiding certain procedures or patients
- Demanding easier shift patterns or shift swaps
- Arrogance masking lack of knowledge
- Leaving work early or showing up late
- Phoning in sick with minor illnesses
- Reliance on alcohol or drugs

These may all be signs of a colleague who is not coping and it is essential that you are aware of these manifestations. As always the key is early intervention and communication to help the individual understand what their behaviour is doing to all members of the team. You need to ask yourself if there is something you could do to help or whether a more senior colleague's input is required. Above all you cannot ignore the problem.

Talking to your supervisor is typically the best first option. They are experienced and are likely to have come across the situation before. Early intervention can prevent more serious events like harm to a patient. Team meetings can be a good way of sharing concerns and problems that everyone has. There are challenging patients as well as challenging colleagues and a collective approach and sharing of what has been said can only help. We all have different ways of working, some of which jar with others in the team who may have been there longer or have more fixed ideas. Talking through the issues in a non-threatening environment is a good way of resolving the conflict before it escalates.

Dealing with your own difficulties

If you are genuinely not coping or have health issues then you should discuss these with your educational supervisor. You may have already included your health issues in the transfer of information form that comes over from your medical school to the foundation school. Reasonable adjustments may already have been made but you need to be clear that your educational supervisor does actually know what is going on.

You may need time off for hospital appointments or referral to occupational health. You may benefit from working less than full time and need career guidance. All of this is available and should be easy to access.

Figure 12.1 Sample discharge letter

Re: Mr Bolt

St Elsewhere and Somewhere Hospitals

Diagnosis
Essential to say up front the diagnosis

Date of admission ....

History of presenting complaint
This may be just agreeing with the original referring letter or it may be the patient was admitted as an emergency without referral by anyone in the patient's own surgery

Social circumstances
Important to place the level of care and support the patient has on the bearing of the diagnosis. For example, lives alone could suggest that he needs further support on discharge. This is an overlooked part of the letter but the ability to see the whole patient as opposed to just the presenting illness makes the future management of the patient much easier and to ensure that they have the correct support

Findings at examination
This may well reveal physical findings that are a new presentation and will need recording in the patient's GP notes

Investigations and results
This is important information for primary care to document in the notes of the patient as it has a bearing on the future management of the patient's condition

Management
What did you actually do to the patient when they were in hospital? What treatments were tried and what was the outcome? What did the patient understand of their condition? Were carers or relatives spoken to and what was their response and understanding?

Current medication including highlighting changes to admission medication
This is a very important part of the discharge letter and one that can cause confusion if not stated explicitly. The future management of the patient depends on a clear statement of the drugs the patient should now be taking, which ones have been stopped and why. You should also note if this is fully understood by the patient or carers

Follow up by hospital
The GP needs to know who has further responsibility for the patient's current illness. This means letting the GP know if the patient has already been given an outpatient appointment or whether this will be sent in the post following discharge. If the patient does not require any hospital follow up then a management plan can be outlined in the letter as to under what circumstances the hospital would be happy to have the patient re-referred. For example, many surgical operations can be followed up by the GP surgery without needing an outpatient appointment

Follow up by primary care
In this part of the letter you can outline any community services that you have referred the patient to. You can suggest a care pathway plan for the patient which may involve district nurse involvement, further blood monitoring at the GP surgery, referral to a local dietician or indeed any of the community services that the GP has access to

Signature
Ensure that your signature is clear at the bottom of the letter or that it is also typed. This is a legal document and will remain in the notes of the patient for the rest of their life. Check the letter before sending off to ensure the information is accurate and clear

This chapter covers the essential components of communication between those professionals who are charged with the care of a patient, whether they be in a primary care or hospital setting. Many would now view the divide between primary and secondary care as artificial. Shared care and care pathways now form a large part of the treatment of patients, particularly those with chronic conditions. Communication within teams and from primary to secondary care is essential to ensure the patient gets the correct treatment and follow-up care.

Written communication

The main areas that you will be responsible for include:
- Discharge letters
- Referral letters, including internal referral in hospital
- Clinic letters informing the GP of the review of their patient

Remember these are the record of the patient's stay or interaction with you or your department. It is the basis on which further treatment may be planned or initiated. You need to ensure that all information is properly recorded. It can and will be used as evidence in court.

It is therefore essential that you have a good understanding of exactly what should be contained within the written document that you are about to produce. It is essential you can:
- Accurately prescribe long-term medication
- Take an active part in discharge planning meetings
- Recognize and record when patients are fit for discharge
- Produce a competent, legible, immediate discharge summary that identifies principal diagnoses, key treatments/interventions, discharge medication and follow-up arrangements

Discharge letters

These should document the original reason for the admission. While that may not cover the final diagnosis it does help place the thinking and the management of the patient within the context of the presenting complaint. A simple template will help you ensure that key elements are not left out. Look at the following very familiar headings (Fig. 12.1):
- Diagnosis
- History
- Examination
- Investigations and results
- Management
- Current medication including changes to admission medication
- Follow up by hospital
- Follow up by primary care

Following this schedule will at least ensure you think about each of the important sections of information that the next health professional will need to continue the care of that patient, safely and effectively. The most important aspects of the letter are what has been diagnosed, how the patient was managed, what the investigations have shown, what the current treatments are and exactly what is now required to follow up and manage the patient. It is also worth adding into the letter what the patient has been told and understands about their condition and future management.

Referral letters and internal referrals

When you work in the community you will have need to refer patients into hospital either as an emergency admission or for a further outpatient opinion. If this is an emergency admission then you will have to speak on the phone to the admitting team. You will need to ensure you can clearly state:
- Presenting complaint

- Name and age of patient
- What you have found on examination
- What you think the diagnosis is
- What you are asking the hospital to do
- If the patient is known to the department
- What is their current medication
- Previous medical history
- Who you are

This should be followed by a letter to the hospital and given to the patient carer or ambulance team as a further record for the admitting team.

When referring a patient for an outpatient appointment you will have clearly more time and access to their records. In addition to the points above you will be able to include:
- Patient's hospital number
- Social circumstances
- Relevant investigations you have already undertaken
- Level of urgency you feel the condition warrants
- What the patient or family understands about the referral

While these may seem like long letters it is essential to be concise and ensure that the relevant information is easy to pick out.

Internal referrals for an opinion from another hospital department are also very common. These are now normally done on a specialty-specific proforma. This ensures that the department gets the information that is also relevant to their management of the patient, e.g. whether the patient is continent or not, their level of mobility.

Clinic letters

Again, when you are in the outpatient department you will have to write back to the GP to let them know what you have done and said to the patient. There is a difference between a follow-up outpatient appointment and a new referral. If this is a follow up you should think about:
- Is the patient presenting any new symptoms?
- Are further investigations needed?
- Does the patient need to be seen again in outpatients or can they be discharged?

This final point is essential as it can be very easy just to offer the patient a further appointment when it is really not necessary and the patient can be managed back in the community. You will need to ensure that you agree with your supervisor that the patient can be discharged.

If this is a new referral then you will have to take a full history, and undertake an examination and investigations pertinent to the presenting complaint. The letter back to the GP should then let them know what you have done for the patient and what further tests may be required. Again, it is essential to let the GP know about the following:
- Preliminary diagnosis
- Further investigations undertaken
- Any immediate change to medication
- What follow up is being done and by whom
- What the patient or carer understands of the process

TOP TIPS

- Be clear in verbal and written communications
- State what you are expecting the referral body to do
- Document any changes to medication
- State whom is responsible for further management of the patient
- Document the patient's understanding of what is happening to them

---

13 Introduction to evidence-based medicine

Figure 13.1 Using PICO to answer a clinical question

Step 1:

ASK an answerable question

Scenario	As an F2 doctor in orthopaedics you admit a man with an established history of alcohol dependence and recent high use for an emergency hip replacement. You are wondering what is the most effective treatment to safely manage the patient's withdrawal from alcohol? Some colleagues suggest diazepam and others suggest chlordiazepoxide.

4-part clinical question	**Patient** Adult man with alcohol dependence
	Intervention(s) Diazepam
	Comparison(s) (if appropriate) Chlordiazepoxide
	Outcome(s) Prevention of alcohol withdrawal symptoms including delirium tremens

Question to be answered	Is diazepam more effective and safer than chlordiazepoxide in the treatment of a man with alcoholdependence who has been admitted for an emergency hip replacement?

	Therapy/aetiology harm √	Frequency	Prognosis	Diagnostic accuracy
Type of question/ study design	• SR of RCTs • RCT • Cohort study • Case-control study • Case series • Expert opinion	• SR of cohort studies • Cohort study • SR of RCTs • Case series • Expert opinion	• SR of diagnostic studies • Diagnostic study • Expert opinion	• SR of surveys • Single survey • Expert opinion

Step 2:

ACCESS (SEARCH FOR) the best AVAILABLE evidence

	Primary term	Synonym 1	Synonym 2	
Structured search strategy	P (alcohol dependence	OR	OR)	AND
	I (diazepam	OR	OR)	AND
	C (chlordiazepoxide	OR	OR)	AND
	O (withdrawal	OR tremens	OR)	AND

*Note: consider truncation for each word and add an *, e.g. child* rather than children*

	Database 1:	Hits	Database 2:	Hits

Key reference	
Key finding	

It is hard to argue with the principle that patient care should be informed by the best available evidence. This chapter covers how to use evidence to inform decisions about patient care or enable patients to make informed decisions about their own care.

What is evidence-based medicine?

Evidence-based medicine (EBM) is the integration of the best available evidence, clinical experience and patient values in patient or clinical decision making. This approach has revolutionized decision making in healthcare. Instead of just relying on reasoning from the basic sciences, EBM demands that your clinical decisions are informed by the best available clinical research data. In other words, evidence showing that a drug *does* work in clinical practice is valued above inferences from basic sciences that a drug *should* work.

Why is it important?

There were two main drivers for EBM:
- The need to manage information overload
- The need to make sure patient care is informed by the best available evidence

With over 2 million articles published each year in 20 000 biomedical journals, it is impossible for busy clinicians to keep up-to-date without competence in EBM. In addition, you will be aware that publication in a scientific journal is no guarantee of study quality. EBM helps you to question 'received wisdom' and constructively appraise research findings to determine whether they are valid, important and applicable to your specific clinical situations.

How to practice EBM – the five steps

EBM can be broken down into five steps, sometimes known as the fives 'As':
1 **A**sk structured clinical questions.
2 **A**ccess the best available evidence.
3 **A**ppraise the evidence.
4 **A**pply the evidence.
5 **A**ssess performance and patient outcomes.

Step 1 – how to ask structured clinical question

Many questions emerge in the course of clinical practice. One model for translating uncertainty into an answerable question is to break it down into four parts known by the acronym, PICO:
Patient
Intervention (or **E** for exposure)
Comparison
Outcome
An example of a clinical scenario and a question formulated using PICO is given in Fig. 13.1.

Step 2 – how to access (search for) the best available evidence

It is clearly impractical to systematically retrieve and critically appraise the primary literature for every question that emerges in clinical practice. Meta-resources (e.g. BMJ Clinical Evidence) present pre-appraised summaries, which address some of the more common clinical questions, and evidence-based guidelines (e.g. NICE, SIGN) are increasingly common.

The best available evidence will depend on the type of question you are asking:

- Questions about treatment (therapy and harm) and what caused a condition (aetiology) are best addressed by systematic reviews (SRs) of randomized controlled trials (RCTs)
- What is likely to happen to a person with a condition (prognosis) is best addressed by a systematic review of cohort studies
- Questions about the diagnostic accuracy of an investigation are best addressed by a systematic review of diagnostic studies
- How common a condition is (prevalence) is best addressed by systematic reviews of surveys otherwise known as cross-sectional studies

Electronic databases such as PubMed, Embase and the Cochrane Library are useful resources for searching the scientific literature:
- PubMed is provided free by the US National Library of Medicine. It is North American focused
- Embase tends to catalogue more European journals
- The Cochrane Library includes the Cochrane Reviews, which are regarded as the gold standard for systematic reviews, and the Cochrane Controlled Trials Register (CCTR). The CCTR contains randomized and controlled trials drawn from sensitive searches of a number of databases including Embase and PubMed

Most electronic databases use Boolean logic (AND, OR, NOT) to combine search terms. If you wanted to find as many of the therapy studies as possible addressing the question in Fig. 13.1, you could combine the outcome terms using the 'OR' term for a comprehensive search.

Step 3 – how to critically appraise the evidence

Critical appraisal addresses three questions:
- Is the research applicable or generalizable to my patient?
- Is it valid?
- Is it important?

Critical appraisal of RCTs and systematic reviews of RCTs is covered in Chapter 14.

Step 4 – how to apply the evidence in practice

The best available evidence is only one factor that should be taken into account for patient or clinical decision making. Clinical considerations such as the severity of the illness and co-morbid risk factors must be considered. When making decisions, you should also draw upon your experience. Decisions are taken in the context of healthcare policy, e.g. what is available in our particular health economy. There may be specific legal considerations that need to be taken into account.

Step 5 – how to assess your performance

Whatever the source of the evidence, the critical step is the last one: the assessment of performance. This is easier described than practised but you must not only evaluate how faithful you were to the first four steps of EBM process but also assess whether your patient has been helped. It may be that a review of the evidence focusing on the care of an individual patient highlights opportunities to improve the care of other patients.

TOP TIPS
- Searching for the evidence can be slow
- Set aside time to search for and review the evidence
- Keep a note of questions arising during your clinical practice
- For therapy questions check guidelines first

Figure 14.1 The GATE frame

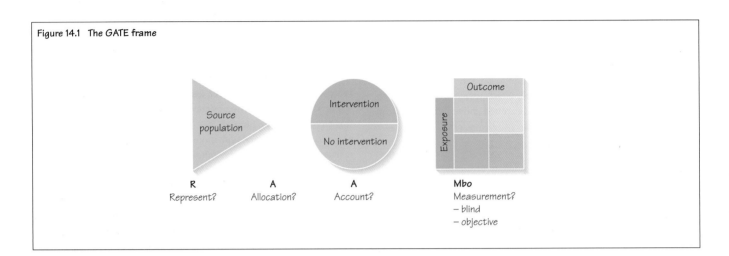

R	A	A	Mbo
Represent?	Allocation?	Account?	Measurement? – blind – objective

Figure 14.2 Effect measures

Term	Definition	How is it calculated?
Control event risk (CER)	The proportion with the event of interest in the control group	$\dfrac{\text{Number of events (controls)}}{\text{Total number in control group}}$
Experimental event risk (EER)	The proportion with the event of interest in the intervention group	$\dfrac{\text{Number of events (intervention)}}{\text{Total number in intervention group}}$
Absolute risk reduction (ARR)	The difference in risk between the control and experimental groups	$ARR = CER - EER$
Number needed to treat (NNT)	The number needed to treat with the intervention to prevent one additional person experiencing the adverse event. Conventionally, the NNT is rounded up	$NNT = \dfrac{1}{ARR}$
Risk ratio (RR)	The risk of experiencing the event in the experimental group relative to the control group	$RR = \dfrac{EER}{CER}$
Relative risk reduction (RRR)	The proportion of events that would have been avoided in the control group had they been allocated the intervention	$RRR = 1 - RR = \dfrac{ARR}{CER}$

Questions about whether a drug or other intervention is effective are best answered by randomized controlled trials (RCTs) or systematic reviews of RCTs. This chapter covers the critical appraisal of RCTs. The critical appraisal of systematic reviews is covered in Chapter 15.

From your reading of the scientific literature, you will be aware that publication in a peer-reviewed journal is no guarantee of quality. To ensure that your clinical decisions are informed by the best available evidence, you must be able to critically appraise and identify the best available evidence.

What is critical appraisal?

Critical appraisal addresses three questions:
1 Is the research applicable to your patient?
2 Is it valid?
3 Is it important?

Is the RCT applicable and valid?

The critical appraisal of RCTs need not be daunting. As you can see in Fig. 14.1, it can be broken down into a triangle, a circle and square, with the acronym RAAMbo. This is known as the GATE framework and can also be applied to other types of research study.

The **triangle** represents how participants were selected for the RCT. Where did the participants come from (source population) and is the sample who participated in the study representative of the source population?

The **circle** is divided into two segments: the total number of those receiving the intervention of interest and the number receiving the comparison (e.g. placebo, another intervention).

The **square** can be broken down into a two-by-two table when considering dichotomous or binary outcomes (event or no event).

Having extracted the key data about the participants, you should consider the potential pitfalls in the design and execution of the study (RAAMbo):

• **R**epresentative asks the question, 'Is your patient sufficiently similar to the participants in this study?' This is also known as generalizability, external validity or applicability
• **A**llocation considers how the participants were allocated to the intervention and comparison groups. Properly conducted RCTs use randomization with allocation concealment. This seeks to reduce the risk of selection bias by achieving balance between the two groups with respect to both known and unknown risk factors. Imbalance between the intervention and comparison group results in confounding, i.e. other reasons for observing differences in the two groups apart from the intervention of interest. Allocation concealment prevents clinicians subverting the process of randomization. This can happen if the clinician knows what the next allocation in the sequence is. It can be avoided when the study uses remote call centres to randomize participants
• **A**ccounted asks whether all participants are still accounted for at the end of the RCT. However, this is rarely the case and typically some participants will withdraw from the study, switch treatment or be lost to follow up. To maintain the integrity of the original allocation, attempts should be made to analyze all participants in the group to which they were allocated. This may mean that you need to make judgements about how to handle drop outs, e.g. last observation carried forwards where you use the last available result for each participant even if they didn't complete the study. Analyzing all participants in the group to which they were originally allocated is known as 'intention-to-treat' analysis. Studies that experience a significant difference in drop outs across the two or more arms are prone to bias
• **M**easurement of outcomes typically requires some subjective judgement and there is a risk that the outcome assessors may apply different thresholds depending on whether the participant was allocated to a particular intervention. Blinding ('**b**') is a strategy to reduce the risk of measurement bias and it is important that the study authors describe who was blinded and how it was achieved. There is less scope to make judgements if the outcome measures are objective ('**o**'), e.g. death

Assuming you are satisfied that any failings in the design or execution of the study are not catastrophic, you can turn your attention to the numbers or importance of the study.

Are the results important?

When dichotomous (event or no event) outcome measures are used, it is possible to calculate measures of effect such as absolute risk reduction (ARR), risk ratio (RR), relative risk reduction (RRR) and number needed to treat (NNT). These terms are described in Fig. 14.2.

The terms ARR and RRR are used when the intervention reduces the risk of adverse events. Absolute benefit increase (ABI) and relative benefit increase (RBI) are more appropriate descriptors when considering positive outcomes.

Is it a poor quality study or a poorly reported study?

Most studies involving large numbers of people rarely go exactly to plan. Even the most perfectly designed study will encounter problems in its execution. It is common for participants to withdraw and no longer be available for follow up.

Mindful that word limits and copy space present researchers and editors with challenges, even the most fundamental information about the conduct of the studies is often omitted. Therefore it is often difficult to judge whether the study is of poor quality or just poorly reported. Sometimes more information is available on the journal's website.

TOP TIPS – HOW TO READ A PAPER IN LESS THAN 15 MINUTES

• Read the title – is it likely to address the question of interest?
• Read the abstract – is the paper applicable to your patient? Does it address your focused clinical question? Does it use an appropriate study design? Having spent no more than a minute, you should be able to make a judgement as to whether the paper is worth more detailed consideration
• Only read the final paragraph of the introduction. The introduction rarely provides any useful information for critical appraisal. But the hypothesis under consideration or the aim of the study is usually described in the final paragraph
• Read the methods and results sections. These provide the data needed to critically appraise the paper
• There may be no need to read the discussion section. Having critically appraised the paper you can come to your own conclusions

Critical appraisal of systematic reviews and meta-analyses

Figure 15.1 Explanation of a forest plot

RR (95% CI random) – a risk ratio (RR) was calculated for each study. The risk ratios are represented graphically by a square with a 95% confidence interval (CI) depicted as a line on either side. If the CI for any study does not cross the line of no effect (in this example RR = 1) then this indicates a statistically significant effect at the 5% level (P <0.05). The numerical results are given in the column to the right

Random – random effects refers to the type of statistical analysis undertaken. An alternative method is a fixed effects model

Weight – a weighted average of the results is used in meta-analysis so that smaller studies exert less influence than larger ones. The relative amount of weighting per study is dependent on the type of analysis (fixed or random)

Comparison: Any antidepressant v placebo (new relapses/participants at risk – any duration of prior treatment)

Outcome: Combined relapse/recurrence (0–12 months)

Study	Antidepressants n/N	Placebo n/N	RR (95% CI random)	Weight %	RR (95% CI random)
Cook 1986	0/7	3/9		0.4	0.18 [0.01,2.98]
Coppen 1978	3/16	5/16		1.7	0.60 [0.17,2.10]
Doogan 1992	24/185	48/110		8.1	0.30 [0.19,0.46]
Feiger 1999	9/65	19/66		4.3	0.48 [0.24,0.98]
Frank (IPT) 1990	2/28	12/26		1.4	0.15 [0.04,0.63]
Frank (MC) 1990	5.25	15/23		3.4	0.31 [0.13,0.71]
Georgotas (NTP) 1989	7/13	7/14		4.2	1.08 [0.52,2.23]
Georgotas (PHZ) 1989	2/16	8/9		1.6	0.14 [0.04,0.52]
Kasper 1999	31/143	78/140		9.9	0.39 [0.28,0.55]
Kishimoto 1994	2/12	13/14		1.7	0.18 [0.05,0.64]
Kupfer 1992	0/11	5/9		0.4	0.08 [0.00,1.21]
Montgomery 1988	23/108	54/112		8.5	0.44 [0.29,0.67]
Montgomery 1993b	11/68	29/67		5.4	0.37 [0.20,0.69]
OADIG 1993	8/33	19/36		4.7	0.46 [0.23,0.90]
Reynolds 1999	13/53	31/54		6.5	0.43 [0.25,0.72]
Robinson 1991	7/31	13/16		4.5	0.28 [0.14,0.56]
Rouillon 1991	140/767	120/374		13.1	0.57 [0.46,0.70]
Rouillon 2000	17/104	26/110		6.2	0.69 [0.40,1.20]
Terra 1998	10/110	24/94		4.6	0.36 [0.18,0.71]
Versiani 1999	29/145	73/141		9.5	0.39 [0.27,0.56]
Total (95% CI)	343/1940	602/1440	◇	100.0	0.42 [0.35,0.49]

Test for heterogeneity chi-square = 30.80 df = 19 p = 0.042
Test for overal effect z = 9.92 p = <0.00001

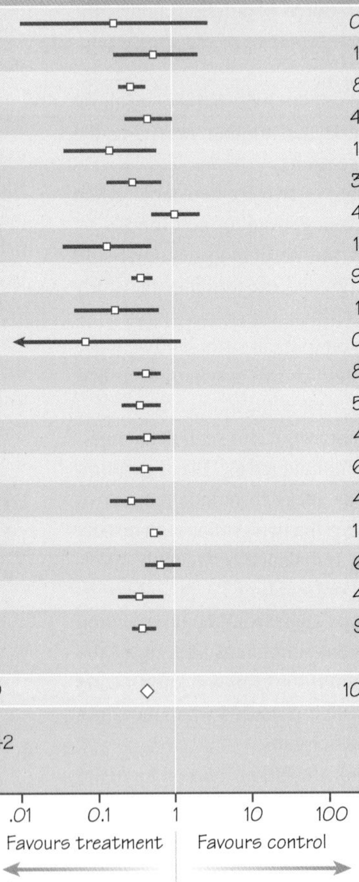

```
        .01     0.1      1      10     100
        Favours treatment  |  Favours control
```

Total (95% CI) – this is the combined estimate for the risk ratio with a 95% CI. It is depicted graphically as a diamond and if it crosses the line of no effect (in the above example RR = 1) the results are not statistically significant at the 5% level

Test for heterogeneity – systematic reviews typically use a chi-squared test for heterogeneity. A P value of less than 0.1 is taken to suggest that there may be underlying heterogeneity. Random effects analyses are more appropriate with a test for heterogeneity P value of <0.1. You can also eye-ball the results – if you cannot draw a straight line through all of the 95% CIs, this would suggest that there is statistically significant heterogeneity

This chapter covers systematic reviews of randomized controlled trials. The example used considers how long patients with recurrent depression should continue on antidepressant treatment.

A good systematic review summarizes all the best available research evidence on a particular topic. Systematic reviews are useful because evidence from a range of different studies with similar results is more compelling than evidence from only one.

Systematic reviews also lend themselves to meta-analysis, i.e. a statistical summary of the results of all of the combinable studies. This combined result provides you with a more accurate estimate of the effectiveness of an intervention and can help guide you make a clinical decision.

The critical appraisal of systematic reviews can be broken down into four steps:
- Question
- Find
- Appraise
- Synthesis

Question – does it ask a clearly focused question?

Systematic reviews seek to summarize the research evidence in response to a focused clinical question. Therefore the first step is to ask, 'Does the systematic review ask a clearly focused clinical question?'

It should be possible to break down the question into four parts: patient, intervention, comparison and outcome (**PICO**):

Patient – adults with recurrent depressive disorder who have responded to acute treatment with an antidepressant

Intervention – continue antidepressant

Comparison – stop antidepressant (and switch to placebo)

Outcome – relapse or recurrence of depression

The question under consideration should guide the review and determine what should be included (inclusion criteria) and what should be excluded (exclusion criteria).

The type of question will determine what type or types of study should be included. Treatment questions are best answered by systematic reviews of RCTs.

Comparing the question addressed by the systematic review with your own clinical question will help you determine whether this systematic review is worth appraising.

Find – did it find all the best evidence?

The systematic review should clearly describe the search terms used. It should provide sufficient information for you to be able to replicate the search (if you had the time!). The search should be comprehensive and take all reasonable steps to track down all the relevant studies.

When considering whether the search was comprehensive, you should check that the reviewers included:
- All possible search terms
- A selection of electronic databases – different electronic databases focus on specific journals so restricting the search to only one database (e.g. PubMed) may miss important articles not indexed on this database
- Articles published in all languages – ideally the study should include articles published in any language. Studies with favourable and statistically significant results are more likely to be published in English-language journals
- Unpublished studies – the reviewers should contact experts in the field to track down unpublished studies. Studies that do not find

favourable or statistically significant results are more likely never to be published

Appraise – were the studies critically appraised?

The reviewers should assess the quality of the identified studies. Only studies that are methodologically sound should be included. For example, when critically appraising RCTs, the reviews should remember RAAMbo:
- Represent
- Allocation
- Account
- Measurement (blind and objective)

It is often difficult to know what the threshold should be for including studies that have methodological flaws. Therefore, reviewers will typically include all RCTs and repeat any analyses excluding studies with methodological issues. This is called a sensitivity analysis.

Synthesis – were the results appropriately combined?

Assuming that it is appropriate to include the studies, the data can be presented as a table describing the results (e.g. how many found a treatment benefit) or they can be combined statistically. Meta-analysis is a statistical technique for combining the numerical results of the included studies.

The results of a meta-analysis are presented as a forest plot. The one shown in Fig. 15.1 is from the systematic review investigating over what period of time the initial benefits of antidepressants are maintained in patients with recurrent depressive disorder.

You should consider whether it is appropriate to combine the results of the identified studies in a meta-analysis. Only studies asking sufficiently similar questions should be combined. In addition you must also be satisfied that the studies are of a sufficiently high quality.

The results of the included studies are presented with their 95% confidence intervals (CIs), i.e. the range of values within which you can be 95% confident the true result lies. If all of the studies were similar, you would be able to draw a straight line through all of the CIs. As you can see, there is some variation, known as heterogeneity, in the RCTs combined in this example. Heterogeneity can be introduced because of variations in the study quality, study populations, interventions, duration of follow up, etc.

The featured meta-analysis attempts to take account of the variation between studies using a random effects statistical model. The summary estimate is presented as a diamond and suggests that continued treatment with antidepressants reduces the risk of relapse in patients with recurrent depressive disorder. As the confidence interval around the summary estimate does not cross the line of no effect (i.e. a risk ratio of 1), the results are statistically significant.

What could you tell your patient?

This systematic review and meta-analysis suggests that 16% of patients with recurrent depressive disorder who continue on antidepressants are likely to experience a relapse within a year compared to 42% who stop treatment. The final decision rests with your patient.

> **TOP TIP**
>
> - There are four steps when critically appraising systematic reviews: question, find, appraise, synthesis

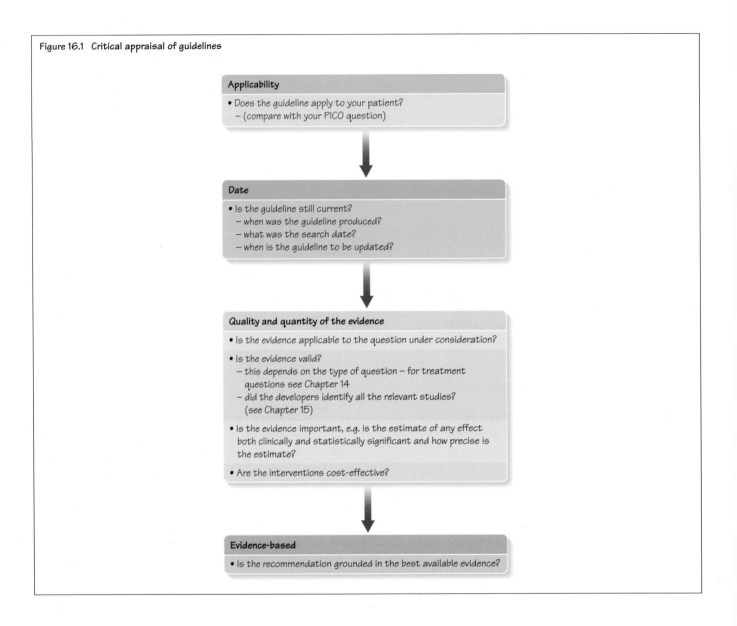

Figure 16.1 Critical appraisal of guidelines

Applicability
- Does the guideline apply to your patient?
  - (compare with your PICO question)

Date
- Is the guideline still current?
  - when was the guideline produced?
  - what was the search date?
  - when is the guideline to be updated?

Quality and quantity of the evidence
- Is the evidence applicable to the question under consideration?
- Is the evidence valid?
  - this depends on the type of question – for treatment questions see Chapter 14
  - did the developers identify all the relevant studies? (see Chapter 15)
- Is the evidence important, e.g. is the estimate of any effect both clinically and statistically significant and how precise is the estimate?
- Are the interventions cost-effective?

Evidence-based
- Is the recommendation grounded in the best available evidence?

This chapter covers the critical appraisal of guidelines and protocols and explores how you can use the recommendations in your clinical practice. Clinical guidelines and protocols are part of day-to-day clinical practice. Good quality guidelines and protocols pull together the best available evidence in response to clearly focused questions, are explicit about the strengths and weaknesses of the underlying evidence and make evidence-based recommendations.

They can help clinicians improve the quality of patient care by reducing unnecessary variation and promoting good practice. However, uncritical use of guidelines and protocols can be harmful as the evidence may not apply to your patient or the recommendations may be flawed.

What is the difference between a guideline and protocol?

Guidelines are systematically developed recommendations to support you and your patients make decisions, e.g. the NICE guideline for the assessment and management of adults with depression. Protocols prescribe what steps should be taken in the care of a patient with a particular condition, e.g. resuscitation algorithm, protocol for alcohol detoxification.

Guidelines are typically developed by national agencies or professional associations and protocols tend to be locally developed (but not always). Both guidelines and protocols should be the product of a systematic review of the evidence.

How to find guidelines and protocols

You should first be clear what question or questions you are seeking to answer. As discussed earlier, the **PICO** (patient, intervention, comparison, outcome) model is helpful when framing your question and guiding your search for the most appropriate guidance.

The first place you should look for guidelines is either NICE (National Institute for Health and Care Excellence) or SIGN (Scottish Inter-Collegiate Guideline Network). Many professional associations (e.g. British Thoracic Society, British Association for Psychopharmacology) often have their own guidelines. In addition, local guidelines and protocols will be available where you work (typically on the intranet).

How to critically appraise a guideline or protocol

There are four components to critically appraising a guideline (Fig. 16.1):

1 Does it apply to my patient?
2 Is the guideline current?
3 Is the evidence underpinning the guideline relevant, valid and important?
4 Is the recommendation based on the evidence?

There are many factors that impact on the validity and importance of the underlying evidence, including the quality of the studies, the quantity of evidence and whether the studies agree. NICE uses a four-point scale to rate the evidence in their guidelines.

High	Further research is very unlikely to change our confidence in the estimate of the effect
Moderate	Further research is likely to have an important impact on our confidence in the estimate of the effect and may change the estimate
Low	Further research is very likely to have an important impact on our confidence in the estimate of the effect and is likely to change the estimate
Very low	Any estimate of effect is very uncertain

Economic analyses typically form part of the evidence under consideration; guidelines consider the affordability of any interventions within a particular health system. Therefore, a guideline is likely to be most prescriptive when the quality and quantity of the evidence is rated as 'high' and the intervention is deemed cost-effective.

Finally, you must consider whether the recommendations are grounded in the evidence and that the patient you are treating is sufficiently similar to the types of patients considered.

How to use guidelines and protocols

By their very nature, protocols tend to prescribe what course of action should be taken when caring for a specific patient. Guidelines provide guidance in the form of recommendations. Both should be grounded in the best available evidence and should have benefited from clinical and patient expert input.

Where protocols exist, they should be the default position for clinical care. As a healthcare professional you are responsible for considering whether the protocol is applicable to your patient. In addition, you must ensure that you enable the patients you are treating to make informed decisions about their care. If you and the patient decide to derogate from the protocol, you should seek advice from a senior colleague and document the reasons for the decision in the patient's notes.

Similarly, where guidelines exist you should consider whether they are relevant to your patient and consider the recommendations in partnership with your patient. The following provides a model for enabling patient decision making:

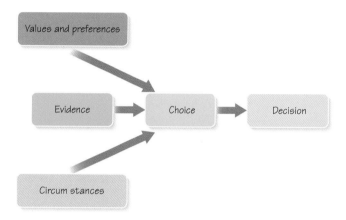

As you will see, the evidence is only one factor in determining a decision. Both patients and clinicians bring their values, preferences and expertise to any decision. In addition, the patient's circumstances (e.g. co-morbidities) will impact on the choices available.

It is important that you are clear that the patient has all the necessary facts and understands them, including the risks and benefits, when considering treatment options (see Chapter 10).

TOP TIPS

- A systematic review should underpin each recommendation or statement
- Ask yourself, 'Is my patient sufficiently similar to the patients considered by the guideline?'
- If you and the patient choose to deviate from a guideline or protocol, documents this clearly in their notes.

17 Running a teaching session and presentation skills

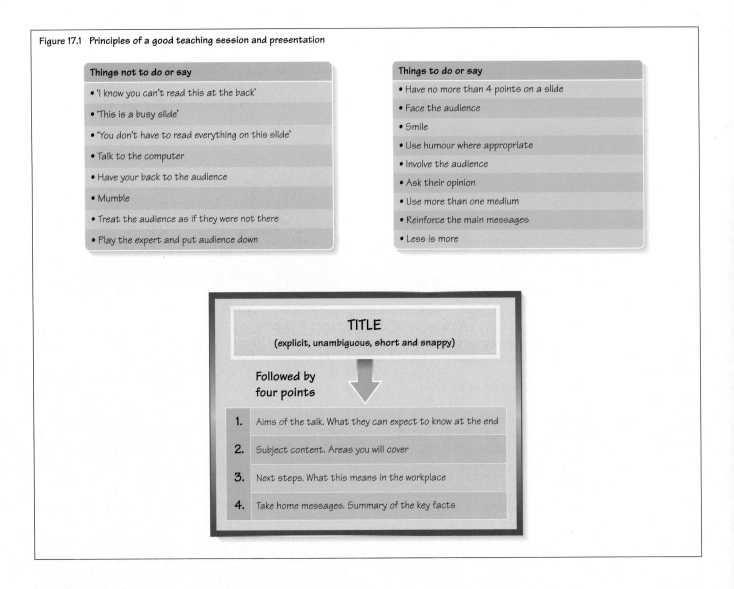

Figure 17.1 Principles of a good teaching session and presentation

Things not to do or say

- 'I know you can't read this at the back'
- 'This is a busy slide'
- 'You don't have to read everything on this slide'
- Talk to the computer
- Have your back to the audience
- Mumble
- Treat the audience as if they were not there
- Play the expert and put audience down

Things to do or say

- Have no more than 4 points on a slide
- Face the audience
- Smile
- Use humour where appropriate
- Involve the audience
- Ask their opinion
- Use more than one medium
- Reinforce the main messages
- Less is more

TITLE
(explicit, unambiguous, short and snappy)

Followed by four points

1. Aims of the talk. What they can expect to know at the end
2. Subject content. Areas you will cover
3. Next steps. What this means in the workplace
4. Take home messages. Summary of the key facts

This chapter covers how to deliver presentations and teaching sessions that support learning.

Throughout your education you will have encountered great and poor teaching. What makes a teaching session or presentation great? Is it one or more of the following?

- Content
- Style
- Interest of subject
- Enthusiasm of presenter
- Skill and knowledge of how to run a great session

You may already have had the opportunity to do a teaching session with other students from a lower year or run one for colleagues on the ward. What principles did you use to underpin the message you were trying to get across?

Maximising learning

The following list gives an aid to how best to maximize the learning opportunity for the students (Fig. 17.1):

1 Arouse and motivate. The first 20 seconds are probably the most important part of your session. Get their attention at the start and you will keep them till the end.

2 Present objectives of the session. Let them know exactly what they should know and understand by the end of the session.

3 Link up with their previous knowledge. You need to build on what students already understand and therefore you need to understand your audience and at what level they function.

4 Communicate clearly what has to be learnt. All too often we try and cram too much information into a session. Be clear. Understand what the top take-home messages are. Less is more!

5 Structure. Give short introductions about the topics to be covered. Scene setters aid audience understanding of what to expect.

6 Activate the learner. Get the learners involved. Make the session interactive.

7 Provide feedback. This is essential to reinforce the session's message and the understanding of the learners.

8 Promote knowledge transfer. Find ways of embedding the knowledge in real life situations that the learner understands and can use. Clinical case discussions are a good example of this.

9 Facilitate retention. Help the learners retain the information by giving them tasks to undertake or provide summaries of the information as a 'take-home message'.

You may not find it easy, at first, to use all these principles in every teaching session and thus you may want to focus on the 'FAIR' principles:

Feedback: this should be realistic, specific, immediate and frequent
Activity: get the student to put the theory into practice
Individualize: plan your session to cater for the audience, not yourself
Relevant: link the new knowledge to what they will practically do on the wards

Choosing the right media

Once you understand the principles that underpin the educational session you want to give, you now have to choose the right medium to get your message across. It is all about ensuring that you maximize the impact of the teaching on the audience. They fall broadly into four headings:

- Print
- Audio
- Audiovisual
- Practical/simulation

The choice of best medium is seldom absolute and you need to consider many factors. Your final choice must take into account the teacher, the learner, the institution and the teaching aim. Consider the following:

- What objective am I trying to achieve?
- Do any of the learning objectives dictate the use of a specific media?
- Am I simply wishing to introduce some interest and variety into the main media of learning?
- Could the use of an alternative media help stimulate discussion and reinforce ideas?

Consider some of the positive attributes of each media.

PowerPoint

This remains the basis for most presentations because it is a visual medium. However, it remains a challenge to get this pitched at the right level. We have all heard the phrase 'death by PowerPoint' and many still fall into the trap. It should be a prop for the talk or presentation, not just an exact copy of what you are going to say. It should allow you to develop the points you want to make, not just in reality replace you as the audience can read it all word for word. The best PowerPoint presentations therefore make use of the following (Fig. 17.1):

- Less on a slide is more
- No more that four points per slide

- Use of illustrations or pictures to make the point
- Humorous cartoons where applicable
- Large font size so anything on the slide can be seen by all
- Clearly stating the aims and objectives on the first few slides so the audience understands what you are trying to get across
- Film clips as appropriate
- Restrict the number of slides to the smallest number that gets the issue across rather than overkill with dozens of slides

Printed material
- Quick to produce
- Requires no additional equipment for use by learner
- Can have feedback built in

Audio
- This of course could now be a blog or MP3
- Conveys emotion well
- Gives real sound and can record real events
- Is relatively cheap
- Can be used as a stimulus for discussion or written exercises

Videotape
- Is able to show movement
- Is useful for observing your own practice
- Lets you use commercial training videos

Practical/simulation
- High learner buy in
- Mimics real life situations
- Allows learner to become competent before using the skill in real life situation
- Allows instant feedback

Length

The problems most presenters face is trying to fit in too much information into each session. The educational theorists tell us that the attention span of an audience is no longer than 20 minutes, yet how often have you ever had a lecture that stopped after that time?

Emphasize key messages

Good teachers know the key messages they are trying to get across in the session. They reinforce them throughout the talk, even checking at the end by getting the audience to summarize what they have learnt to ensure congruence. Finally, they leave further reading or work for the participants to do to expand on the subject rather than have busy slides.

TOP TIPS

- Engage the audience immediately
- Key messages are essential, detail is not
- Use a medium supportive of your message
- Interact with the audience
- Check their understanding of what you are saying
- Finish with the take home message(s)

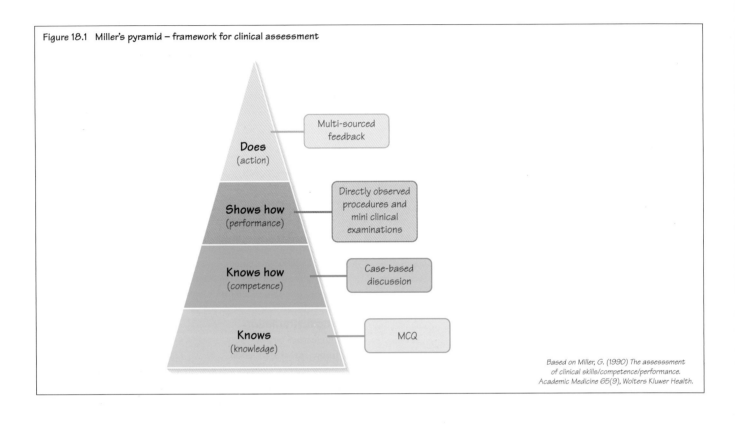

Figure 18.1 Miller's pyramid – framework for clinical assessment

Does
(action)

Multi-sourced feedback

Shows how
(performance)

Directly observed procedures and mini clinical examinations

Knows how
(competence)

Case-based discussion

Knows
(knowledge)

MCQ

Based on Miller, G. (1990) The assessment of clinical skills/competence/performance. Academic Medicine 65(9), Wolters Kluwer Health.

This chapter covers the principles of assessment and feedback as they apply to you in the foundation programme. Chapter 3 discussed what assessments you need to complete to provide evidence of satisfactory performance. You will also be responsible for assessing others in the team and providing constructive feedback. Therefore it is essential that you have a good understanding of the principles that underpin assessment and feedback.

Assessment methodology

Assessments can be either formative or summative. Since summative assessments are likely to be done by your own educational supervisor on you to check your progress, it is more likely that you will be involved in formative assessments with peers or medical students. Improvement in an individual's performance will only occur if regular assessment leads to constructive feedback. This can happen with formative assessment when the individual knows that the purpose is to improve their performance rather than an end stage summative mark for the task at hand.

Assessment tools

There are several assessment tools used in the foundation programme (see Chapter 3). You will be familiar with the following:
- Multi-source feedback (team assessment of behaviour, TAB)
- core procedures
- clinical supervisors end of placement report
- educational supervisors end of placement report
- educational supervisors end of year report

The key principle of assessment is to have a good understanding of the tools you are being asked to use. Fully understanding the purpose is also essential to being able to undertake the procedures or the interaction under discussion. The other major factor is to understand the standard against which you are making a judgement as to the competence or otherwise of both yourself and others that you might be assessing. What constitutes a pass? What constitutes a fail and what would give cause for real concerns?

Miller's pyramid of clinical competence (Fig. 18.1)

This is a very good way of looking at what you are both trying to achieve and observe when assessing the competence of individuals. It divides into sections that enable an individual to demonstrate growing improvement to the level at which they competently perform:
- Knows – fact gathering
- Knows how – through case presentation
- Shows how – demonstration of learning via simulation
- Does – through direct observation in the work place

All of this is underpinned by the individual's knowledge skills and attitudes that take them from novice to expert. A clear understanding of these principles will help your own performance and your ability to assess others within the work place.

Assessment demonstrating cause for concern

You have a duty to patients to ensure that they are treated appropriately, safely and respectfully. If you feel a peer or more junior colleague shows a failing in their dealing with patients as demonstrated when you undertook an assessment on them, then you have to know how best to proceed.
- Be clear what the issue is
- Discuss your concerns with the individual
- Form an action plan with them if its a minor error
- Follow up with a repeat assessment
- Let your supervisor know what you have done and found
- Ask for further support for the individual from their supervisor
- Make a written record of the event

You cannot walk away from a clinical problem that has arisen or may arise from the actions of an individual that could in any way compromise the patient, the individual or the clinical team. Assessments are there to help review progress and improve performance.

Feedback

In any assessment process it is important to be able to give feedback in a timely and constructive way. The benefits of the assessment process may be lost if the message is not delivered in a way that the recipient can positively understand.

Principles of feedback

If you are undertaking assessments then you have to be trained to give feedback. It should be:
- Specific
- Timely
- Factual
- Given in an appropriate environment
- Not rushed
  Also:
- Allow time for further clarification
- Be available for follow up by the recipient

Giving feedback

It is likely that you will be required to assess and provide feedback to medical students and colleagues. This should be done sensitively and in a suitable environment. Always be specific and try to offer alternatives:
- 'I wonder if you have tried … ?'
- 'How else might you have done that … ?'
- 'Perhaps you could have … ?'

It is equally important not to be dishonestly kind. The information you are giving can have a direct effect on the future performance of the receiver and therefore to patient care.

One model for giving constructive feedback is outlined below:
1 Clarify any points of fact.
2 Ask the learner what went well.
3 Discuss what went well, adding your own observations.
4 Ask the learner what went less well.
5 Discuss what went less well and agree next steps.
6 Get them to summarize the learning points from the discussion.

The best feedback is given close to the actual incident and done in a non-judgemental way in an appropriate and private setting. The object is to improve the performance of the individual not to further demoralize them.

Feedback is a skill and it takes time to master but will be used for the rest of your career.

TOP TIPS

- Be clear what you are trying to assess
- Use the appropriate tools for the assessment
- Know the expected standard that person should achieve
- Make sure feedback is timely
- Be honest in your feedback

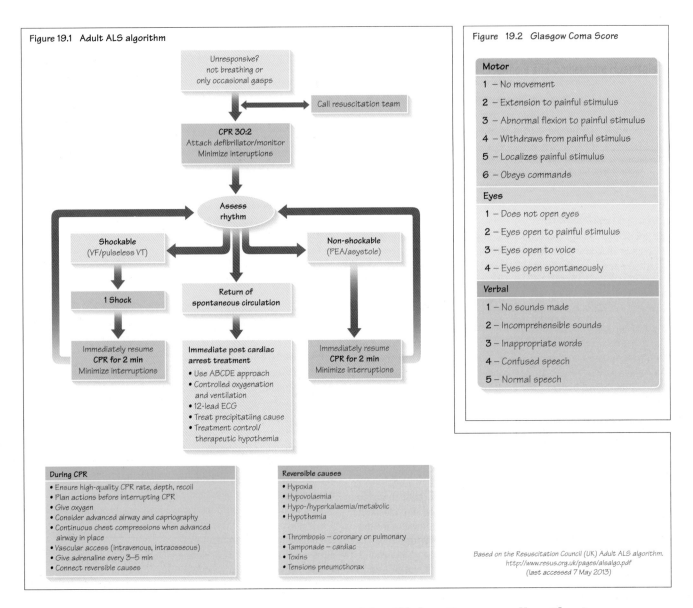

Figure 19.1 Adult ALS algorithm

Unresponsive?
not breathing or
only occasional gasps

Call resuscitation team

CPR 30:2
Attach defibrillator/monitor
Minimize interuptions

Assess rhythm

Shockable
(VF/pulseless VT)

Non-shockable
(PEA/asystole)

1 Shock

Return of
spontaneous circulation

Immediately resume
CPR for 2 min
Minimize interruptions

Immediate post cardiac
arrest treatment
• Use ABCDE approach
• Controlled oxygenation
  and ventilation
• 12-lead ECG
• Treat precipitatiing cause
• Treatment control/
  therapeutic hypothemia

Immediately resume
CPR for 2 min
Minimize interruptions

During CPR
• Ensure high-quality CPR rate, depth, recoil
• Plan actions before interrupting CPR
• Give oxygen
• Consider advanced airway and capriography
• Continuous chest compressions when advanced
  airway in place
• Vascular access (intravenous, intraosseous)
• Give adrenaline every 3–5 min
• Connect reversible causes

Reversible causes
• Hypoxia
• Hypovolaemia
• Hypo-/hyperkalaemia/metabolic
• Hypothemia

• Thrombosis – coronary or pulmonary
• Tamponade – cardiac
• Toxins
• Tensions pneumothorax

Based on the Resuscitation Council (UK) Adult ALS algorithm.
http://www.resus.org.uk/pages/alsalgo.pdf
(last accessed 7 May 2013)

Figure 19.2 Glasgow Coma Score

Motor
1 – No movement
2 – Extension to painful stimulus
3 – Abnormal flexion to painful stimulus
4 – Withdraws from painful stimulus
5 – Localizes painful stimulus
6 – Obeys commands

Eyes
1 – Does not open eyes
2 – Eyes open to painful stimulus
3 – Eyes open to voice
4 – Eyes open spontaneously

Verbal
1 – No sounds made
2 – Incomprehensible sounds
3 – Inappropriate words
4 – Confused speech
5 – Normal speech

This chapter covers the acute assessment of adult patients who have become unwell. It provides a system for safely and efficiently treating life-threatening problems before senior help arrives.

The assessment of acutely ill patients is a common task for foundation doctors. Without a logical approach this can be a challenging, stressful and even frightening experience.

When someone becomes acutely unwell, the priority is to establish likely causes for the deterioration, and begin treatment that will deal with these problems. It is not necessary to come to a firm diagnosis, and it is often appropriate to initially give treatment for more than one potential cause. Some patients are too unwell to be managed by just one doctor; in these circumstances remain calm, and have the confidence to ask a senior colleague to assist.

Identifying the unwell patient

Often the most difficult part of treating a sick patient is recognizing they have become unwell. Patients can tolerate acute physiological insults remarkably well and early warning signs are easily overlooked or misinterpreted. Repeated assessment of the patient and measurement of the vital signs helps identify worsening trends as they emerge.

The general 'end-of-the-bed' eyeball assessment can be surprisingly accurate. Patients who look unwell usually are unwell, though the reverse is not always true. It is helpful to say aloud when you think someone is unwell: this will often prompt nurses (and other doctors) into action.

Many hospitals use 'early warning score' charts to record vital signs. As the values become physiologically worse, the rising warning score triggers a request for a doctor to review the patient.

Many patients who suffer an 'unexpected' cardiac arrest have had significantly abnormal vital signs for hours, if not days, before the eventual cardiac arrest. Do not ignore subtle changes in the vital signs, particularly if there is a trend in the wrong direction. Drugs may mask these early changes; for example a patient who takes β-blockers may have a normal heart rate despite significant blood loss. Remember that apparently normal values for one patient may be grossly abnormal for another; beware the hypertensive patient with 'normal' blood pressure!

Approaching the acutely ill patient

When you are asked to see a sick patient, go to their bedside before spending time looking through the case notes. Always ensure you can actually see and hear them! Turn on the lights and turn off televisions, radios and other distractions. Important clinical signs like cyanosis or stridor are easily missed in dark or noisy rooms.

Establish the background to the patient's deterioration. Ask someone to find the case notes while you assess the patient. Often the notes will tell you what has already been discussed with the patient and their relatives, for example if resuscitation should be attempted in the event of cardiac arrest.

Initial assessment

The ABCD (Airway, Breathing, Circulation, Disability) approach is easy to remember, and helps identify and correct the most potentially life-threatening problems in the order they should be dealt with. Treat each problem below as you identify it; don't be tempted to fully examine the patient before starting any treatment.

Airway

If your patient cannot maintain their airway and simple airway manoeuvres do not correct this immediately, call the cardiac arrest team and begin Advanced Life Support (ALS) (Fig. 19.1).

From the end of the bed, noisy breathing – or no breathing at all – suggests the airway is in danger. Try a chin-lift and jaw-thrust manoeuvre, and consider inserting a nasopharyngeal or oropharyngeal airway adjunct.

Patients with a Glasgow Coma Score (Fig. 19.2) of 8 or less require airway protection, and should be reviewed urgently by a doctor with airway skills, usually an acute medicine physician or anaesthetist.

Patients who are speaking are protecting their airway.

Breathing

Is the patient breathing? If not, call the cardiac arrest team and begin ALS.

Count the respiratory rate, auscultate the chest and check the oxygen saturations. Give high-flow oxygen via a non-rebreathing mask initially, regardless of whether or not they have chronic obstructive airway disease. The patient is much more likely to come to harm from acute hypoxia than from retained carbon dioxide. Only when the oxygenation improves should you reduce the inspired oxygen concentration.

Patients with a low respiratory rate may be intoxicated with drugs, (prescribed or illicit) including opiates and benzodiazepines. Consider giving naloxone, which antagonizes opiates. Flumazenil, which reverses benzodiazepines, should be used with caution as it may precip-itate seizure activity that the benzodiazepine was previously suppressing. Remember that naloxone and flumazenil both have short half-lives, so may wear off before the opiate or benzodiazepine is eliminated from the blood. Repeated doses or infusions may be necessary, especially when the patient has renal or hepatic dysfunction (which delays drug metabolism). Note that naloxone is not licensed for infusion, so this should first be discussed with a senior doctor.

Circulation

Check the carotid pulse and the blood pressure. If there is no palpable carotid pulse, immediately summon the cardiac arrest team and begin ALS.

If the patient is hypotensive, or has a downwards trend in the last few blood pressure readings, assume they are hypovolaemic initially. Give a bolus of fluid and if the blood pressure responds, give further fluid. If not, consider alternative causes such as cardiogenic shock, sepsis syndrome or drug effects. Consider why the patient might be hypovolaemic, and seek urgent help if the cause is not immediately obvious.

Hypovolaemia is the commonest reason for shock, and in the short term it is usually safer to give fluid than to withhold it, irrespective of other medical problems. If the patient has advanced heart or kidney failure, seek senior advice as soon as you begin administering fluid, as too much fluid may become harmful over time.

Disability

Always check the blood glucose level. This can be checked quickly with a bedside monitor, but send blood for a formal laboratory glucose measurement too. If the bedside glucose is less than 3.5, the patient needs sugar. If they are conscious, give a sugary drink. If unconscious, give 10% or 50% IV dextrose. If there is not a fast clinical response (within 1–2 minutes), or if intravenous access is proving very difficult, give IM glucagon. (Glucagon is usually stored in a fridge.)

Assess the Glasgow Coma Score and check the core temperature. If the patient is hypothermic, consider a warming blanket and/or warmed intravenous fluids. Remember that sepsis syndrome can manifest as low as well as high temperatures, especially in older people.

When should I call for help?

You should never be criticized for asking for help with a sick patient. If the cause for your patient's deterioration is unclear; if they do not respond quickly to your treatment; or you are at all unsure what to do, immediately summon senior help. If the nurse who is helping you with a sick patient suggests contacting your seniors for advice, it is usually wise to follow their advice.

TOP TIPS

- Always investigate abnormal vital signs
- Never be afraid to ask for senior help
- A cardiac arrest call will summon urgent senior help; your patient is more likely to survive if you do this before they arrest!
- The ABCD approach helps you quickly identify and manage the most serious problems while waiting for senior help to arrive

Figure 20.1 Prescription chart

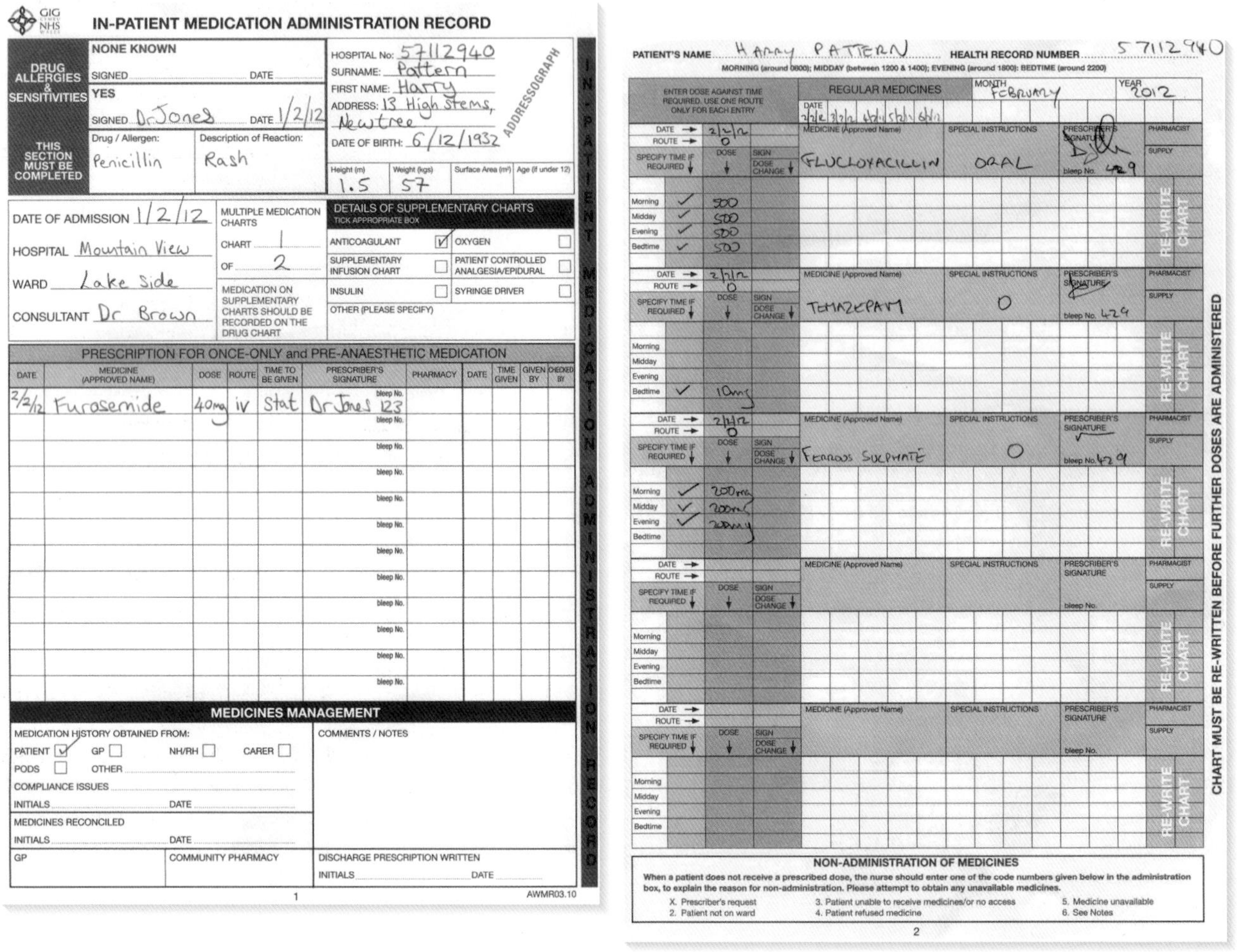
IN-PATIENT MEDICATION ADMINISTRATION RECORD

DRUG ALLERGIES & SENSITIVITIES: NONE KNOWN — SIGNED — DATE; YES — SIGNED Dr Jones DATE 1/2/12

THIS SECTION MUST BE COMPLETED — Drug / Allergen: Penicillin; Description of Reaction: Rash

HOSPITAL No: 57112940
SURNAME: Pattern
FIRST NAME: Harry
ADDRESS: 13 High Stems, Newtree
DATE OF BIRTH: 6/12/1932
Height (m): 1.5 — Weight (kgs): 57 — Surface Area (m²) — Age (if under 12)

DATE OF ADMISSION 1/2/12
HOSPITAL Mountain View
WARD Lake Side
CONSULTANT Dr Brown

MULTIPLE MEDICATION CHARTS: CHART 1 OF 2

DETAILS OF SUPPLEMENTARY CHARTS (TICK APPROPRIATE BOX): ANTICOAGULANT ✓; OXYGEN; SUPPLEMENTARY INFUSION CHART; PATIENT CONTROLLED ANALGESIA/EPIDURAL; INSULIN; SYRINGE DRIVER; OTHER (PLEASE SPECIFY)

PRESCRIPTION FOR ONCE-ONLY and PRE-ANAESTHETIC MEDICATION

DATE	MEDICINE (APPROVED NAME)	DOSE	ROUTE	TIME TO BE GIVEN	PRESCRIBER'S SIGNATURE	PHARMACY	DATE	TIME GIVEN	GIVEN BY	CHECKED BY
2/2/12	Furosemide	40mg	iv	Stat	Dr Jones 123					

MEDICINES MANAGEMENT
MEDICATION HISTORY OBTAINED FROM: PATIENT ✓ GP NH/RH CARER PODS OTHER
COMPLIANCE ISSUES — INITIALS — DATE
MEDICINES RECONCILED — INITIALS — DATE
GP — COMMUNITY PHARMACY — DISCHARGE PRESCRIPTION WRITTEN — INITIALS — DATE
COMMENTS / NOTES

PATIENT'S NAME Harry Pattern — HEALTH RECORD NUMBER 57112940
MORNING (around 0800); MIDDAY (between 1200 & 1400); EVENING (around 1800); BEDTIME (around 2200)

REGULAR MEDICINES — MONTH February — YEAR 2012

DATE	ROUTE	MEDICINE (Approved Name)	DOSE	SPECIAL INSTRUCTIONS	PRESCRIBER'S SIGNATURE
2/2/12	O	FLUCLOXACILLIN	500 (Morning, Midday, Evening, Bedtime)	ORAL	bleep No. 429
2/2/12	O	TEMAZEPAM	10mg (Bedtime)	O	bleep No. 429
2/2/12	O	FERROUS SULPHATE	200mg (Morning, Midday, Evening)	O	bleep No. 429

CHART MUST BE RE-WRITTEN BEFORE FURTHER DOSES ARE ADMINISTERED

NON-ADMINISTRATION OF MEDICINES
When a patient does not receive a prescribed dose, the nurse should enter one of the code numbers given below in the administration box, to explain the reason for non-administration. Please attempt to obtain any unavailable medicines.
X. Prescriber's request; 2. Patient not on ward; 3. Patient unable to receive medicines/or no access; 4. Patient refused medicine; 5. Medicine unavailable; 6. See Notes

Figure 20.2 Yellow adverse reaction chart

YellowCard — It's easiest to report online at www.yellowcard.gov.uk — MHRA

SUSPECTED ADVERSE DRUG REACTIONS

PATIENT DETAILS: Patient Initials: H.P. Sex: M. Ethnicity: White British. Weight if known (kg): 80. Age (at time of reaction): 82. Identification number: 5712940

SUSPECTED DRUG(S)/VACCINE(S): Flucloxacillin; Batch 769A; Route O; Dosage 500mg; Date started 2/2/12; Date stopped 2/2/12; Prescribed for Skin infection

SUSPECTED REACTION(S): Urticarial rash, increasing problems breathing, swollen extremities. Treatment: I.V. steroids. Outcome: Recovered ✓
Date reaction(s) started: 2/2/12. Date reaction(s) stopped: 4/2/12
Do you consider the reactions to be serious? Yes / No — Involved or prolonged inpatient hospitalisation ✓

OTHER DRUG(S) (including self-medication and complementary remedies): Did the patient take any other medicines in the last 3 months prior to the reaction? Yes
Furosemide; Route O; Dosage 40mg; Date started 1/1/12; Date stopped on going; Prescribed for CCF

Additional relevant information: Known CCF. Admitted in failure. Skin infection noted on admission. Treatment started. Swabs sent.

REPORTER DETAILS: Dr. Deen, University Hospital Northampton; Postcode NN4 2PU; Speciality: Cardiology; Date 5/2/12

CLINICIAN (if not the reporter)

Please attach additional pages if necessary. Send to: FREEPOST YELLOW CARD (no other address details required)

 The Foundation Programme at a Glance, First Edition. Stuart Carney and Derek Gallen. © 2014 John Wiley & Sons, Ltd. Published 2014 by John Wiley & Sons, Ltd.

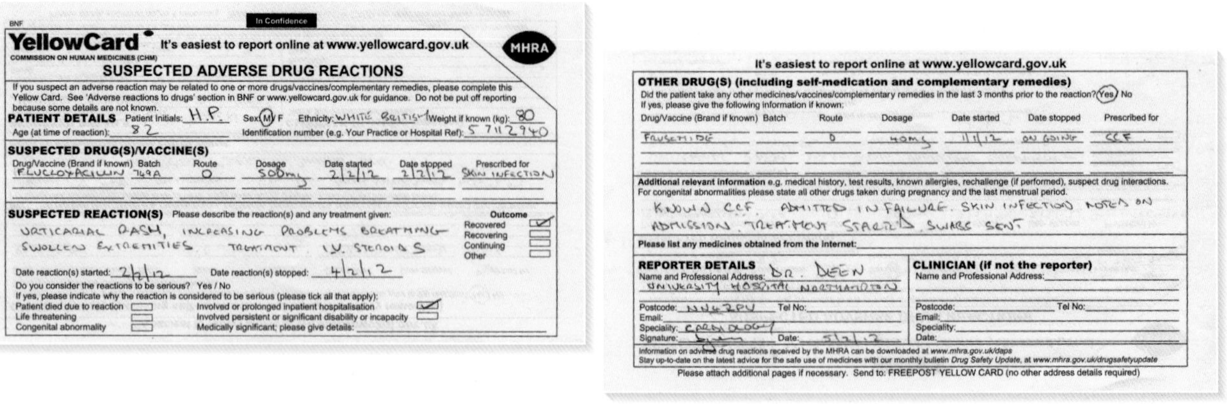

Drug therapy remains the mainstay of treatment for patients and is also responsible for the largest numbers of medical errors. Many of these errors are minor and have no damaging effects on patients but others have lasting, severe consequences. While all grades of doctors make prescribing errors, there are simple measures that can be put into place to prevent this occurring. The increased use of polypharmacy to treat co-morbidities requires a balance to be struck between known side effects and interactions against the overall benefit and acceptability to patients.

This chapter covers the principles of rational prescribing, compliance and drug reactions.

First steps

Take an accurate drug history. This may seem obvious, but should include:
- Current drugs and dosages
- Allergies
- Any self-medications the patient has taken
- Recent drugs that have been stopped, e.g. steroids
- Homeopathic remedies
- Compliance
- Drug misuse and alcohol consumption

It is also worth documenting what the patient understands about the drugs that they have been prescribed and their compliance to the regimen. Have they arrived in hospital with full tablet boxes that should have been used long ago? This may alter your thinking on whether they will actually take the treatment prescribed when they are discharged.

Prescribing

The drug chart (Fig. 20.1) is a legal record of the treatment the patient has received or is receiving. You have to ensure that you write legibly and accurately to ensure that the pharmacist and the nursing staff that administer the drugs are giving the correct drug, formulation and dosage. Many hospitals now have computer-based prescribing which automatically goes to the pharmacy. This has the added advantage that the computer can immediately alert to drug interactions and to pre-scribing dose errors. If a kardex system is used then the unique patient identifier should be at the top, together with any known allergies, ahead of the actual prescribing lines. Consider:
- The *BNF* should be your bible
- The pharmacist is your friend and a great source of information
- When in doubt, ask

Treatment

The first question you have to ask yourself is whether a drug treatment is required at all. It is essential that you do not make things worse. Polypharmacy often contributes to acute episodes of illness, including delirium.

The second question, when a patient is on multiple medications, is how many of these can be rationally and safely stopped? It can be very easy to add therapies rather than fundamentally reviewing the reasons for the original prescriptions. For example, a patient presenting in pain may be prescribed co-codamol. This causes constipation, so a laxative is prescribed. As the patient is now not sleeping a night sedative is prescribed. It can therefore quickly escalate into all subsequent drugs being prescribed to offset the side effects of the original tablet. If the pain had been properly assessed in the first place then alternatives to drugs may have been better, e.g. physiotherapy.

Compliance

It is all very well getting the right diagnosis and indeed the correct and appropriate drug treatment, but you have to maximize the chances of the patient wanting to take the medication. Consider the following:
- How many times a day does the medication need to be taken?
- By what route is the medication taken?
- Is it easy to swallow?
- Does it taste nice?
- Does it make the patient feel better or worse immediately after taking?
- Does the patient know why they are taking the medication?

It seems obvious that the best way to get a patient to take the medica-tion is to have the simplest regimen, the easiest route, a palatable format and no side effects. It is also important that the patient understands that they must complete the course of medication not just stop when they feel better, or if the medication should be taken indefinitely.

External effects on prescribing

Age, weight, genetic susceptibility, hepatic impairment, and renal impairment can have an effect on the bioavailability of the drug in the system. Simple, normally prescribed drug dosages can have wildly different titres in the body depending on these factors and they can lead very easily to both undertreatment and toxicity if they are not taken into account. You should also consider the impact of cultural and religious beliefs, pregnancy, breast feeding and allergies.

Drug reactions

It is likely at some time in your professional life that you will prescribe a drug that the patient reacts too. These reactions may be classified as:
- Known and documented side effect of the drug
- Unknown and allergic reaction to the drug

As previously discussed, when you prescribe a drug there is a balance between the good it will do the patient and the possible side effects that may occur. Nausea is a common side effect of many medications but the benefits of the treatment may well outweigh the symptom. However, a severe reaction or anaphylaxis should always be reported to the Medicines and Healthcare Products Regulatory Agency (MHRA). This can be done by the 'yellow card scheme' (Fig. 20.2).

What to report
- All reactions to new drugs (black triangle in *BNF*)
- Reactions in elderly
- Reactions in children
- Reactions in pregnancy
- Life threatening (anaphylaxis) reactions
- Fatal reactions
- Any reactions where you think the drug was the cause of the problem

---

TOP TIPS
- Remember prescribing is a legal record
- Love your *BNF*
- The pharmacist is your friend
- Always consider if a drug is necessary
- Review polypharmacy to rationalize intake
- Consider optimal frequency, route and formulation
- When in doubt, ask
- Write all dosages in full
- Avoid abbreviating micrograms or milligrams

Figure 21.1 Guidance for medical record keeping

1. Requirements of an adequate entry in the case notes

- Legible handwriting
- Date and time of entry
- Relevant clinical details
- Signature
- Printed name and grade

2. SOAP

- **S**ubjective assessment of symptoms
- **O**bjective measurements including vital signs, blood test results
- **A**ssessment or working diagnosis
- **P**lan of action

4. Common pitfalls in medical record keeping

Remember that your documentation in the case notes may be the only record of your clinical interaction with that patient. It may be assumed that you had access to the full set of case notes when documenting your review, so be sure to mention 'no old notes' if they were not available when you saw the patient. If you do not document something it is assumed to not have occurred, so it is important to clearly record negative as well as positive findings in the history and examination. It is also worth recording the location of your review if it did not occur in your normal ward, e.g. if the patient is being accommodated in an outlying ward during a bed shortage

3. Improve your record keeping

- When you meet a patient for the second time, read your previous entry in the notes – can you reconstruct the clinical encounter based upon your entry?
- Have you documented a clinical impression or working diagnosis?
- Ask a colleague to read your entry in the notes; is your handwriting really legible?
- Before documenting a subjective opinion, consider whether you would be comfortable making the same statement to the patient, or reading it aloud in court

 The Foundation Programme at a Glance, First Edition. Stuart Carney and Derek Gallen. © 2014 John Wiley & Sons, Ltd. Published 2014 by John Wiley & Sons, Ltd.

This chapter covers medical record keeping. It includes guidance for making effective entries in the notes, and explains some of the less obvious details about medical records (Fig. 21.1).

Why keep medical records?

Good medical record keeping is an essential part of good patient care. The record describes clinical encounters, is a compendium of past investigations and results, and facilitates continuity of care as the patient interacts with different health professionals. The medical record is also a legal document. It forms the basis of any investigation into the care a patient has received, whether for clinical research, insurance or legal reasons.

What is included in medical records?

Any information about a patient forms part of their medical record, even if it is not physically stored within their paper case notes. This includes handwritten notes, entries on computer databases, electronic or printed photographs, correspondence between health professionals, and laboratory and other investigation results.

Who contributes to medical records?

Doctors, nurses and other allied health professionals should record every interaction with every patient. Notes are usually kept in a single paper or electronic case notes file for that patient. Some departments have their own separate record, with a short summary placed in the main case notes. For example, a cardiac catheterization laboratory might place a one page summary of angiography findings into the case notes, but keep a full set of images and technical findings within a separate cardiology record.

What information should be recorded?

The medical record should contain sufficient information so that readers can reconstruct your consultation and avoid duplicating tests. This facilitates continuity of care as the patient meets different doctors and allied health professionals over one or more clinical episodes. Always record the relevant positive and negative findings, your clinical impression and plan of action having seen the patient. If you do not document something it will be assumed later that you did not consider it; e.g. if you do not document the clinical absence of meningism it is assumed you did not specifically look for this when you examined the patient.

Good records help you approach difficult clinical situations, e.g. when meeting a critically ill patient (and their relatives) for the first time in the middle of the night. It is very helpful to know what has already been discussed and decided prior to your meeting. Notes should also describe significant co-morbidities, allergies and so on – crucial information when a patient is obtunded and unable to communicate with you.

What should not be recorded in the notes?

Only objective, factual information should be recorded, with each entry legibly written, dated, timed and signed. When subjective opinions are

necessary these should never include sarcastic remarks or personal insults about the patient or their relatives. Only record statements you would be willing to make directly to the patient, or read aloud in a court. Patients and their representatives are entitled to access their record; one unfortunate comment can undo many years of hard-earned trust.

Do not make ambiguous statements in the notes. A common mistake is to use abbreviations. A neurologist might understand 'MS' to mean 'multiple sclerosis', while a cardiologist could interpret the same statement as referring to 'mitral stenosis'.

Each patient should have their own individual record, and it should only contain information about them. For example, if a secure e-mail message is used to discuss multiple patients, that message would form part of each patient's medical record, which they are legally entitled to view. This effectively breaches each of the patient's confidentiality.

Confidentiality

All records must remain confidential at all times. Paper notes should be stored securely, and computerized records password protected. Portable electronic storage devices, e.g. USB sticks or DVDs, must be encrypted and password protected. If it is necessary to share clinical information with a colleague, e.g. in a referral letter, then only relevant information should be included.

Do not share your computer passwords with colleagues. Most computerized systems include 'audit trails' tracking the records you have accessed. If your account is used to access records of patients not under your care, this is effectively a breach of confidentiality.

Who can view medical records?

- Medical records are primarily for the use of doctors, nurses and allied health professionals
- Legal authorities including the courts, police or lawyers may also view case notes to investigate a patient's care
- Administrators may also access notes to file results and clinical correspondence; they too are bound by confidentiality rules
- Only relevant parts of notes should be accessible; e.g. dieticians might not necessarily need to see psychiatry records
- Patients or their representatives have the right to view their record; this can only be withheld if there is a genuine risk of harm to the patient or others by disclosing information
- Notes can never be withheld because of inappropriate or offensive remarks made about the patient or relatives

TOP TIPS

- Remember every part of a medical record is a legal document
- Never document anything you would not be prepared to read out and defend in court
- All notes should enable colleagues to reconstruct your consultation with the patient, and avoid duplicating previous investigations

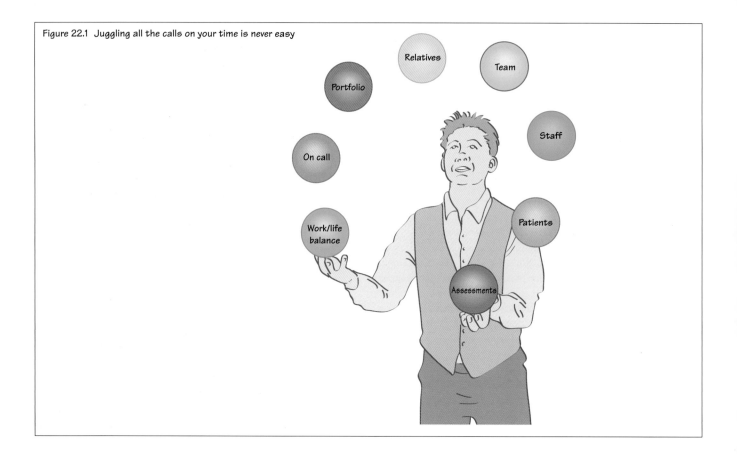

Figure 22.1 Juggling all the calls on your time is never easy

This chapter covers tips on how to best use your time to reduce your stress and get the most out of your day. There are never enough hours in the working day and perhaps there never will be. However, the better you are at managing your time the better the care you will be able to give to your patients.

> A doctor with poor time management skills is going to feel under greater stress and this, in turn, will effect his relationship with patients, ward staff and his own team. (Gallen & Buckle 1997)

Inefficient time management has a knock-on effect not only for you but for the rest of the team. It also prevents you from looking after yourself. If you continually finish late how do you get time for meal breaks? What is the effect on your personal life and friends and family?

Starting as a foundation doctor is a daunting time because the list of jobs that need to be done can seem endless (Fig. 22.1). The first step is to acknowledge that time management is an important skill to develop and consider the following:
- Where do you feel the pressure of time the most?
- Are you doing something that could be delegated?
- Does the organizational set up of the ward make optimal use of your time (are you left waiting for others to help you undertake procedures)?
- Can you learn anything from the way others approach tasks?

- Did you get tips from the outgoing F1 doctor on how to manage workload?

The overriding skill is therefore to be able to **prioritize**.

List writing can be a good step to sorting out how your day will pan out. Decide what is urgent and what is important; there is a difference. A patient may need an urgent blood cross-match before they can get to theatre. A second patient may need their INR check that day – it is important but not urgent. However, do not forget that important issues become urgent if left too long!

How can I maximize my time?
Ward rounds
These are important for consolidating the treatment that patients require and deciding what further procedures, interventions, tests or therapy changes are going to be undertaken. You need to ensure you are aware of any changes to your patients' treatment, so have a printed list of the patients to hand. Use this as your record and checklist for the work you will need to do that day. If further investigations are required on any of your patients, write the forms out during the round when you are not presenting the case to the consultant or registrar. Write the changes to the patients' treatments in the notes as you proceed on the round. Agree amongst your team who will record and write as the round

progresses so all available forms and notes are completed. This will save time and they will be fresh in your memory. If a patient is to be discharged, again use the computer immediately the round ends to sort the discharge drugs. This will speed up the process, release a bed and allow the patient to get home quicker.

Preoperative assessments

There should be a simple template that outlines all you need to do for each patient. Use this checklist to ensure nothing is forgotten. It seems obvious but prioritize the patients who are to be operated on first. Ensure those that need a cross-match are also top of your list of jobs to do. Inform your senior colleagues if you find anything new at the preoperative assessment that may affect the operation, e.g. on examination of a woman admitted for a breast lumpectomy, you find more than one lump.

Ward work

This is where you have to make the most of your organizational skills. You have your list of jobs that you want to undertake that day, but be clear that this will be interrupted. You can help yourself by letting the nursing staff know what you are planning to do and in what order. You can also let them know a time at which you will be available for any work they may need you to do, e.g. signing drug charts. This may help them to not interrupt you every time they are trying to prioritize their own work at the expense of yours! Understand the working timetable of the ward.

- When do blood forms need to be in by for the phlebotomist to collect?
- What is the normal discharge time for patients?
- How long does it take to get patients' discharge drugs back to them?
- When is visiting time for you to see relatives of patients?
- What time do patients go down to theatre in the morning and afternoon?
- When are senior staff available to help you with your assessments?
- What time do your teaching sessions start?
- When do the nursing staff change shift and so are unavailable to help you during handover?

A good understanding of how others work and their timings will also help guide you through the working day.

On call

This is a time that may well stretch your organizational skills to the maximum. This is because of the unpredictable nature of the workload. However, there are things that you can do to help navigate this difficult part of the working week:

- Being on call with your own team (this helps)
- Having a specific role (taking admissions from A&E or wards)

- Knowing whom to contact for help
- Knowing your consultant's home number if he is not on the shift
- Knowing how to access investigations out of hours
- Let the nurses know when you will come to their ward so they know to wait and not bleep you
- Use free time to get the patients' notes up to date and organize information for the morning handover
- Prioritize your work
- Ensure you get enough breaks, food and drinks. It will make you more efficient if you are well hydrated

Protected time

It is not just the time taken to see patients and do the paperwork that needs to be addressed. You will have to undertake audits, get your multi-source feedback, assessments and supervised learning events done, and log them onto the portfolio. Is there any time in your normal working day that is protected or are you considered to be available to anyone and everyone because you carry a bleep? Protected time can and should exist within every working day but you may have to be proactive in finding it! All too often this is the part of the day that is neglected by foundation doctors. They just don't feel any of the time is their own.

- Your teaching sessions should be bleep-free
- Use time when others are not available as your free time, e.g. when the nurses are handing over at the change of shift
- Let the staff know you are doing assessments and how long these will take
- Cross cover with another foundation doctor
- Discuss with your educational supervisor how best to protect your time
- Discuss and learn from your peers how they cope

Finally, do not forget or undervalue 'thinking time' – there can be little time for thinking in a busy job but you need time for this. It should be viewed as time invested, time to step back, refocus and think laterally.

TOP TIPS

- Learn to prioritize tasks
- Ask previous job holders how they managed
- Make sure you have proper drink and food breaks
- Don't forget to ask for help

Reference

Gallen, D.D. & Buckle, G. (1997) *Top Tips in Primary Care Management*. Blackwell Science, Oxford.

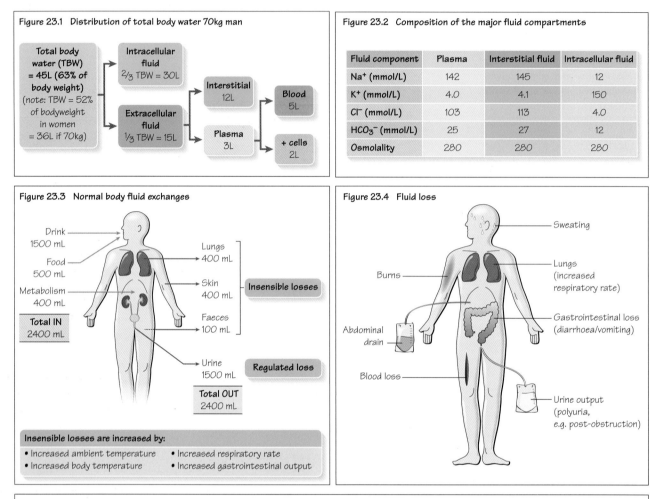

Figure 23.1 Distribution of total body water 70kg man

Total body water (TBW) = 45L (63% of body weight) (note: TBW = 52% of bodyweight in women = 36L if 70kg)

- Intracellular fluid 2/3 TBW = 30L
- Extracellular fluid 1/3 TBW = 15L
  - Interstitial 12L
  - Plasma 3L
    - Blood 5L
    - + cells 2L

Figure 23.2 Composition of the major fluid compartments

Fluid component	Plasma	Interstitial fluid	Intracellular fluid
Na^+ (mmol/L)	142	145	12
K^+ (mmol/L)	4.0	4.1	150
Cl^- (mmol/L)	103	113	4.0
HCO_3^- (mmol/L)	25	27	12
Osmolality	280	280	280

Figure 23.3 Normal body fluid exchanges

Drink 1500 mL
Food 500 mL
Metabolism 400 mL
Total IN 2400 mL

Lungs 400 mL
Skin 400 mL
Faeces 100 mL } **Insensible losses**

Urine 1500 mL } **Regulated loss**

Total OUT 2400 mL

Insensible losses are increased by:
- Increased ambient temperature
- Increased body temperature
- Increased respiratory rate
- Increased gastrointestinal output

Figure 23.4 Fluid loss

- Sweating
- Lungs (increased respiratory rate)
- Gastrointestinal loss (diarrhoea/vomiting)
- Urine output (polyuria, e.g. post-obstruction)
- Blood loss
- Abdominal drain
- Burns

Figure 23.5 Composition of the commonly available replacement fluids

Electrolyte/crystalloid solutions	Colloid solutions
Normal saline: 0.9% NaCl in water = 154 mmol/L Na^+ and Cl^-	**Human albumin solution:** 4.5% albumin solution (derived from pooled donor blood)
5% dextrose: 50 g/L glucose in water (effectively this is equivalent to water)	**Artificial colloids:** Gelatin based, e.g. haemaccel, gelofusin Starch-based, e.g. hydroxyethyl starch, pentastarch
Dextrose-saline: 0.18% NaCl (30mmol/L) and 40 g/L glucose	**Blood:** whole blood or packed cells
Ringer's lactate: 0.6% NaCl, 0.25% Na lactate, 0.04% KCL, 0.27% CaCl (130 mmol/L Na^+, 4 mmol/L K^+, 28 mmol/L lactate, 1.5 mmol/L Ca^{2+})	

Figure 23.6 Impact of infusion on individual fluid compartments

Type of fluid	Extracellular		Intracellular 30 L	Useful in	Not useful in
	Intravascular plasma 3 L	Interstitial 12 L			
Blood 1 L	1000 mL	0	0	Acute blood loss	Salt and/or water loss
Normal saline 1 L	200 mL	800 mL	0	Salt and water loss and sepsis	Burns (use colloid)
5% dextrose 1 L	66 mL	267 mL	667mL	Water depletion (i.e hypernatraemia)	Volume depletion/ blood loss

This chapter covers the management of patients with perturbations in their fluid balance. It outlines the management of patients who require fluids to be prescribed and also patients who are fluid overloaded.

Normal body fluids

The distribution, composition and exchange pathways of body fluids are shown in Figs. 23.1, 23.2 and 23.3, respectively.

Abnormalities of fluid balance

Abnormalities of fluid balance can be broadly divided into states of volume depletion and volume overload. In either situation the outcome can be compromise of organ perfusion.

The volume state is determined by the total body sodium content. Volume depletion implies a reduction in the total body sodium, while volume overload implies an increase in the total body sodium content. It is also important to note that there is no relationship between a patient's volume state and their serum sodium concentration since sodium and water balance are independently regulated. A patient's volume state can only be determined by clinical examination, and no conclusions about volume state can be drawn from a serum sodium concentration.

Assessment of the volume state

Assessment of the volume state is based purely on the clinical history and examination.

Volume depletion

History Patients should be asked about:
- Sources of fluid loss: diarrhoea, vomiting, blood loss, diuretic use
- Any decrease in oral fluid intake
- Symptoms of volume depletion: thirst, postural dizziness, reduced urine output

Examination The signs of volume depletion include:
- Resting or postural tachycardia
- Postural hypotension or supine hypotension if volume depletion is severe
- Reduced jugular venous pressure
- Dry axillae and oral mucous membranes
- Decreased skin turgor (less reliable in the elderly)

Volume overload

History Patients should be asked about:
- A background of relevant disease: heart failure, liver disease/cirrhosis, nephrotic syndrome, kidney failure
- Symptoms of volume overload: swelling of legs or face, exertional breathlessness, orthopnoea, paroxysmal nocturnal dyspnoea

Examination The signs of volume overload include:
- Peripheral oedema (or sacral oedema in bed-bound patients)
- Hypotension or hypertension (depending on the underlying cause)
- Elevated jugular venous pressure
- Gallop rhythm (3rd and/or 4th heart sound)
- Bi-basal fine inspiratory crackles of pulmonary oedema
- Pleural effusions
- Ascites

Management of abnormalities of fluid balance

Volume depletion

The approach to the management of the fluid depleted patient is:
1 Identify the nature of the fluid loss (blood, insensible losses, gastrointestinal loss) (Fig. 23.4).

2 This will help guide the choice of replacement fluid.
3 Estimate the amount of fluid loss (change in body weight, volume state examination, observation charts) and the quantity of ongoing fluid loss.
4 Measure the serum sodium concentration. This will tell you the relative amounts of salt and water and will help guide the choice of replacement fluid. A relative excess of water is indicated by hyponatraemia, and a relative water deficit by hypernatraemia.
5 Select the most appropriate replacement fluid.
6 Infuse fluid at a rate that will restore organ perfusion rapidly, reassess volume state frequently and adjust infusion rate according to response.

Choice of intravenous fluid

In most volume-depleted patients, intravenous fluids are administered. The composition of the commonly available replacement fluids are shown in Fig. 23.5.

In choosing the appropriate fluid replacement, it is critical to identify the nature of fluid loss and also to understand the fate of fluids when they are infused.
- **Blood and colloids**. These remain in the intravascular compartment. Use in situations of blood or plasma loss (e.g. burns)
- **Normal saline**. Saline remains in the extracellular fluid compartment and is distributed proportionately between the intravascular and interstitial compartments. Use in states of volume depletion, i.e. reduced total body sodium
- **5% dextrose**. Since this is water, it distributes proportionately through all fluid compartments. Use in water-depleted patients, i.e. hypernatraemia

The impact of infusion of 1 L of these various fluids on the volume of the individual fluid compartments is shown in Fig. 23.6.

Also note that 5% dextrose and dextrose-saline are hypotonic fluids and if given to volume-depleted patients significant hyponatraemia will develop since the water load cannot be excreted due to baroreceptor-mediated release of antidiuretic hormone (ADH).

Administration and monitoring of fluid replacement

Volume-depleted patients are at risk of end-organ damage caused by reduced perfusion, e.g. acute kidney injury. The aim of therapy is therefore to restore organ perfusion as rapidly as possible. Therefore prescribe fluids to be rapidly infused as a bolus. For example, 500 mL of normal saline infused over 15 minutes.

It also important to recognize that overaggressive fluid repletion can result in pulmonary oedema, particularly in the elderly and those with heart or kidney failure. Therefore, the clinical response needs to be assessed regularly. In high-risk cases, invasive monitoring (e.g. of central venous pressure) may be appropriate.

Boluses of fluid can be repeated until clinical parameters indicate restoration of volume state, i.e. normalization of pulse, blood pressure and jugular venous pressure, and restoration of urine flow.

Once the volume state is corrected, the rate of fluid infusion should be slowed to account for ongoing losses only (see 'Maintenance fluids').

Volume overload

In volume-overloaded patients, total body sodium is increased. This is usually due to renin/angiotensin/aldosterone-mediated renal sodium retention caused by circulatory compromise in heart failure, cirrhosis and nephrotic syndrome, or failure of sodium excretion in renal failure.

It is important to identify the underlying cause and correct where possible.

Treatment of the volume-overloaded patient comprises restriction of dietary sodium intake (to less than 80 mmol/day) and enhancement of urinary sodium excretion using diuretics, particularly loop diuretics (e.g. furosemide/frusemide). Diuretics are far more effective when used in combination with salt restriction. Patients with renal failure may be diuretic-resistant and require dialysis treatment, particularly when pulmonary oedema is present.

Maintenance fluids'

Very often foundation doctors are asked to prescribe maintenance fluids for their patients and this is often a source of confusion. In prescribing fluids consider:

- What a normal person generally requires
- What additional fluid/electrolyte requirements are present (e.g. excess fluid loss due to diarrhoea, enteric drainage, polyuria after relief of urinary obstruction)

Normal daily requirements for an adult are:

- Sodium 50–100 mmol/day
- Potassium 40–80 mmol/day
- Water 1.5–2.5 litres

Add to this an estimate of excess fluid loss taking into account an estimate of the electrolyte content of this lost fluid.

This prescription needs regular review since the clinical situation will change. These fluids can be given orally, via a nasogastic tube or intravenously depending on the clinical situation.

TOP TIPS

- Assess a patient's fluid balance using a combination of their history, examination and hospital fluid charts
- If the patient has evidence of fluid depletion, prescribe a bolus of fluid and promptly review the response
- The type of fluid you give the patient should match their fluid losses/ongoing needs
- Never prescribe fluids repeatedly without first reviewing the patient (not their blood tests or charts)
- In patients with fluid overload, make sure they have a response to diuretics and ensure they are salt restricted

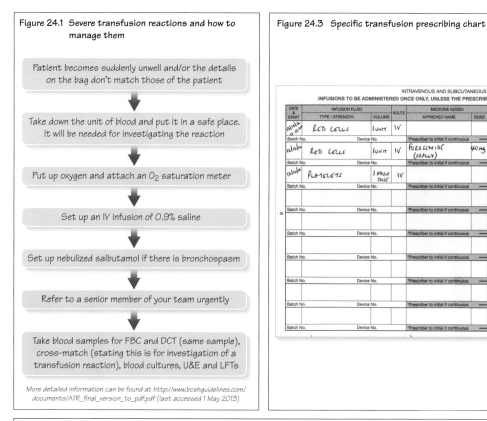

Figure 24.1 Severe transfusion reactions and how to manage them

Patient becomes suddenly unwell and/or the details on the bag don't match those of the patient

↓

Take down the unit of blood and put it in a safe place. It will be needed for investigating the reaction

↓

Put up oxygen and attach an O₂ saturation meter

↓

Set up an IV infusion of 0.9% saline

↓

Set up nebulized salbutamol if there is bronchospasm

↓

Refer to a senior member of your team urgently

↓

Take blood samples for FBC and DCT (same sample), cross-match (stating this is for investigation of a transfusion reaction), blood cultures, U&E and LFTs

More detailed information can be found at http://www.bcshguidelines.com/documents/ATR_final_version_to_pdf.pdf (last accessed 1 May 2013)

Figure 24.3 Specific transfusion prescribing chart

Figure 24.2 IV transfusion prescribing chart

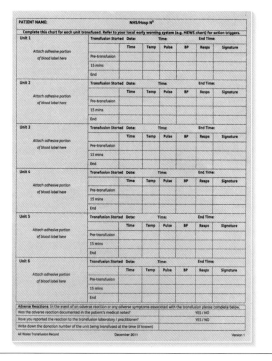

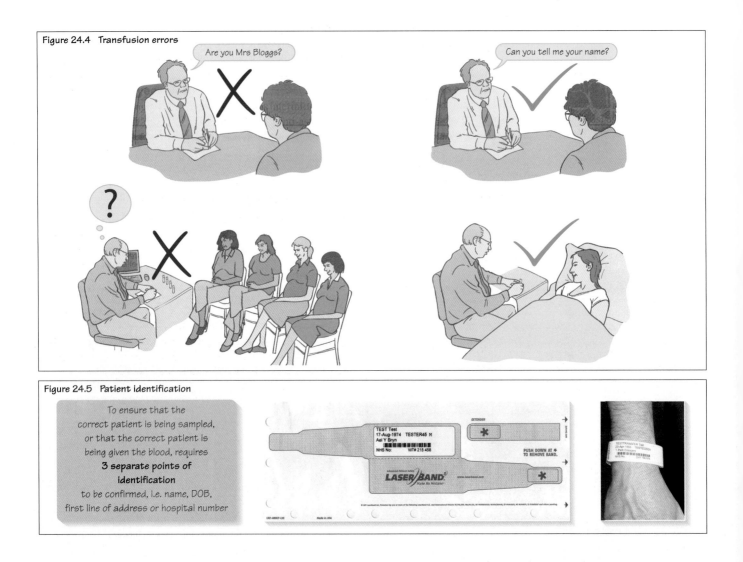

Figure 24.4 Transfusion errors

Figure 24.5 Patient identification

To ensure that the correct patient is being sampled, or that the correct patient is being given the blood, requires **3 separate points of identification** to be confirmed, i.e. name, DOB, first line of address or hospital number

This chapter covers the main issues in prescribing and administering blood products safely. It includes an overview of the risks of transfusion as well as the more common transfusion reactions and their management.

Blood transfusion

The most common type of transfusion is that of red cells. Red cells are given to treat anaemia or for bleeding when the rate of loss could be life threatening. Less often patients require platelets, most commonly as a result of cancer treatment, and for the prevention or treatment of bleeding. Finally, patients can require fresh frozen plasma (FFP) and cryoprecipitate when they have clotting abnormalities.

Risks of transfusion

Blood transfusion in the UK is generally safe and getting safer. Between 1996 and 2009 results from a national reporting scheme (SHOT UK) suggested that only 2/100 000 transfusion episodes are associated with a major morbidity or death (Taylor *et al.* 2010). Also it showed that the complication rates are falling. However, when blood transfusion does go wrong it can be catastrophic and 125 patients are reported to have died either directly from or partly due to transfusions between 1996 and 2009.

The top four complications responsible for almost 80% of events are:
1 Acute lung injury: this is usually seen in the ITU setting where patients are given FFP. It is caused by plasma from female donors who have developed HLA antibodies in pregnancy.
2 Incorrect blood component transfused: the causes include sampling the wrong patient, laboratory errors and putting up the blood on the wrong patient.
3 Acute transfusion reactions: these are allergic reactions.
4 Transmitted infections: recent figures show that viral infections are now almost unheard of and the commonest problem is bacterial contamination.

Other complications are very rare.

Managing transfusion reactions

Acute transfusion reactions are common and it will not be unusual to be called by the nursing staff to see a patient because they have developed a temperature or rash whilst receiving a transfusion. **The first thing to do is to STOP the transfusion whilst you assess the situation.**
1 Check that the details on the transfusion bag match the patient's details. If they do not match then assume this is an ABO-incompatible transfusion.

2 If details match, the patient is comfortable and talking normally:

• and the problem is a **rash** this is likely to be a **mild allergic reaction**. Prescribe chlorpheniramine 10 mg slow IV injection and restart transfusion at a slower rate (but not exceeding a total infusion time of 4 hours)

• and the problem is a **mild fever**, i.e. less than 1.5°C increase, this is likely to be a **mild acute transfusion reaction**. Prescribe paracetamol 1 gm and restart the transfusion at a slower rate (as above)

3 If the patient is unwell with rigors, hypotension, shortness of breath, and bone, muscle, chest or abdominal pain then this is a major reaction and could be due to a severe allergic reaction, ABO incompatibility, bacterial contamination or a haemolytic reaction. Acute lung injury is unlikely in a ward setting. Differentiating these conditions may take time but the acute management is the same (Fig. 24.1).

Staff in the blood bank will advise you on further investigation.

Prescribing blood products

Blood products are prescribed on the IV infusion section of the drug chart (Fig. 24.2) or on a specific transfusion chart (Fig. 24.3).

Important things to know are:

• Transfusions out-of-hours are more likely to lead to errors. Transfusions should wherever possible be completed within the normal working day

• Red cells should generally be given over 2 hours (unless the patient is actively bleeding)

• Red cells should not be given over more than 4 hours and if the blood is still running at 4 hours it should be discarded. This is because it will begins to haemolyze at room temperature

• Most patients can tolerate blood 2 hourly unless they have moderate to severe heart failure or are very elderly. Oral diuretics can be prescribed (Fig. 24.3)

Avoiding transfusion errors

Incompatible blood transfusion is the second most common transfusion complication and can be fatal. The chance of error can be significantly reduced by carrying out patient identification properly (Fig. 24.4). Also, patients with haematological diseases may require special blood products; always let the blood bank know if the patient has a blood disease.

Sampling

1 First complete the transfusion request form.

2 Take the form to the patient's bedside and ask them their identification details. **DO NOT** ask them questions to which they can only answer yes or no as this has been shown to lead to errors. Check the patients' identity bracelet (Fig. 24.5) against the request form. Three points of identification (name, DOB, first line of address or hospital number) must match.

3 Take the blood sample and label it by hand at the bedside. **DO NOT** pre-label as this has been also shown to lead to errors.

4 Attach the sample to the request form at the bedside.

5 DO NOT sample more than one patient at a time.

Setting up a transfusion

Take the unit for transfusion to the bedside and ask the patient their identification details. **DO NOT** ask them questions to which they can only answer yes or no. Check the patient's identity bracelet against the request form. Three points of identification (name, DOB, first line of address or hospital number) must match.

In the unconscious patient check the details on the form or unit for transfusion against the identity bracelet.

Errors are more likely to occur in the emergency setting where doctors are under pressure to not 'follow procedure'. It is exactly this setting where it is most important to follow these steps.

TOP TIPS

• Always ask open questions when identifying a patient
• If a patient is unconscious always check the patient identity bracelet to confirm identification
• Always label samples at the bedside
• The first step in managing a transfusion reaction is to stop the transfusion
• If you are uncertain always ask for help from a senior doctor

---

Reference

Taylor, C. (ed.), Cohen, H., Mold, D., Jones, H. *et al.* on behalf of the Serious Hazards of Transfusion (SHOT) Steering Group (2010) *The 2009 Annual SHOT Report*. www.**shot**uk.org/wp-content/uploads/2010/07/SHOT2009.pdf (last accessed 1 May 2013).

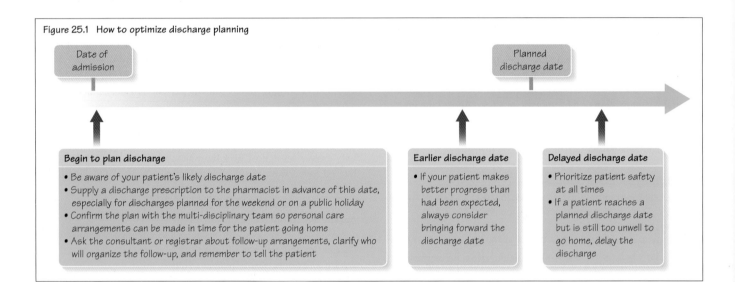

Figure 25.1 How to optimize discharge planning

Date of admission

Planned discharge date

Begin to plan discharge

- Be aware of your patient's likely discharge date
- Supply a discharge prescription to the pharmacist in advance of this date, especially for discharges planned for the weekend or on a public holiday
- Confirm the plan with the multi-disciplinary team so personal care arrangements can be made in time for the patient going home
- Ask the consultant or registrar about follow-up arrangements, clarify who will organize the follow-up, and remember to tell the patient

Earlier discharge date

- If your patient makes better progress than had been expected, always consider bringing forward the discharge date

Delayed discharge date

- Prioritize patient safety at all times
- If a patient reaches a planned discharge date but is still too unwell to go home, delay the discharge

This chapter covers the process of planning patients' discharge from hospital. It explains your part in this process with tips for making it as smooth as possible for you and your patient (Fig. 25.1).

Why is discharge planning important?

Patients should only occupy acute hospital beds when there are medical reasons for inpatient care. Non-medical reasons can often delay discharge, e.g. installation of equipment in the patient's home. These delays expose patients to increased risk of hospital-acquired infections, and reduce the hospital's capacity to admit new acute inpatients.

What is discharge planning?

Patients are usually admitted to hospital for investigations or treatment, with the intention of discharging them once this is complete. Planning the discharge in advance ensures logistical and follow-up arrangements are in place when the patient is ready to go home, and reduces preventable re-admission to hospital.

Discharge planning includes estimating a likely discharge date; considering what other arrangements are needed to support this (e.g. personal care services or district nurse appointments in the community); and organizing follow up.

What is the foundation doctor's role in discharge planning?

As a ward-based doctor you are well placed to liaise between nurses, allied health professionals, patients, relatives and other doctors. You can update the team on your patient's progress and suggest how realistic a discharge date seems. Your overview of the patient helps the rest of the team anticipate and manage potential delays to discharge, such as a need for district nurse follow up.

You will usually be responsible for writing a discharge prescription, which tells the general practitioner about the admission and provides the patient with new medication to take home. The hospital pharmacy will need a few hours notice to dispense medication, and at weekends or on public holidays this may not be possible. Controlled drugs, or dispensing into a dosette box or similar device, will take longer. It is important to work closely with the clinical pharmacist to ensure discharge prescriptions are available in advance of the discharge date. Take care to avoid mistakes if the medication list changes close to the discharge date.

How is a discharge planned?

Discharge planning begins before elective admissions, and at the time of emergency admissions. Simple actions make a big difference. For example, day-surgery patients may not realize that sedation will render them unfit to drive themselves home; by warning about this before admission they can make arrangements to be collected by a friend. This simple advice avoids an overnight hospital stay.

A detailed social history during the admission clerk-in also assists discharge planning. Does the patient live independently at home? Are they dependent on carers visiting several times daily? Personal care services often require 24 hours or longer notice to restart before a patient can be discharged home.

The medical problem that caused the admission will often influence the discharge arrangements. A stroke may render a previously independent patient reliant upon personal care services. The patient who cannot manage at home with a full personal care package might need assessment for placement in supported accommodation. This process can take weeks or months, so should be started when it becomes apparent it is needed.

Discharge planning is usually very straightforward. Occasionally the process can be complicated because of the logistics of coordinating home care, new equipment in the home or geographical difficulties. There may be a hospital discharge team who can help you with these cases. Patients with complex medical needs might also benefit from referral to the local geriatrics service.

Early supported-discharge teams

Patients with chronic illness often need hospital admission when their condition flares. In the past they would be observed in hospital for a lengthy period to ensure their symptoms settled. Many hospitals now have specialist early supported-discharge teams to help these patients. These teams act as a bridge between hospital specialists and recently discharged patients in the community. A specially trained nurse, physiotherapist or occupational therapist regularly visits the patient at home for a period after leaving hospital. This allows safer, earlier discharge from hospital, with a means of prompt specialist involvement if they do not recover as expected.

Specialty-specific nurse-led services can be highly effective in facilitating quick discharges and avoiding preventable admissions to hospital. Heart failure liaison nurses visit patients with heart failure to titrate diuretics and other drugs, balancing heart failure, renal failure and fluid overload. Respiratory early supported-discharge nurses can supply nebulizers and ensure patients continue to improve when they return home from hospital following an exacerbation of chronic obstructive pulmonary disease, among other conditions.

Who can discharge a patient?

• The medical team looking after a patient usually decides when the patient can be discharged from hospital
• A senior nurse can often discharge patients who have had low-risk, elective procedures. Usually there are objective discharge criteria (e.g. normal vital signs and have eaten a meal) which patients must meet before they are allowed home
• Any doctor or registered nurse can delay or cancel a discharge if the patient is not well enough to go home

---

TOP TIPS

• Discharge planning starts with the decision to admit the patient to hospital – either as an emergency, or electively in the future
• Involve other members of the multidisciplinary team
• Consider using early supported-discharge teams
• Plan ahead and anticipate problems before the discharge date
• You can bring forward or postpone the discharge date if the clinical situation changes

---

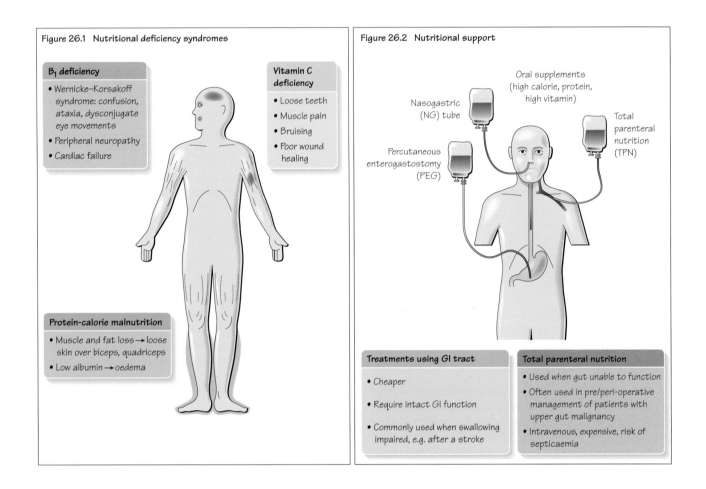

Figure 26.1 Nutritional deficiency syndromes

B₁ deficiency
- Wernicke–Korsakoff syndrome: confusion, ataxia, dysconjugate eye movements
- Peripheral neuropathy
- Cardiac failure

Vitamin C deficiency
- Loose teeth
- Muscle pain
- Bruising
- Poor wound healing

Protein-calorie malnutrition
- Muscle and fat loss → loose skin over biceps, quadriceps
- Low albumin → oedema

Figure 26.2 Nutritional support

Oral supplements (high calorie, protein, high vitamin)

Nasogastric (NG) tube

Total parenteral nutrition (TPN)

Percutaneous enterogastostomy (PEG)

Treatments using GI tract
- Cheaper
- Require intact GI function
- Commonly used when swallowing impaired, e.g. after a stroke

Total parenteral nutrition
- Used when gut unable to function
- Often used in pre/peri-operative management of patients with upper gut malignancy
- Intravenous, expensive, risk of septicaemia

The extent of malnutrition in hospital inpatients is often underestimated. Many diseases lead to anorexia and a reduction in calorific intake, and this is especially relevant when placed in the context of the increased nutritional requirements resulting from the catabolic state of malignant or inflammatory disease.

This chapter covers the impact on the patient of nutrition deficiencies and the indications for specific diets. It is important to understand the nutrition status of every patient when they present to the hospital setting. It can have a profound effect on the rate of recovery of the patient, the bioavailability of drug therapies and indeed may even be the reason they have been admitted.

Specific malnutrition (vitamin and mineral deficiencies)

Acute vitamin deficiency is much more frequent with the water-soluble vitamins (particularly vitamin B_1 (thiamine) and vitamin C) (Table 26.1), rather than those that are fat soluble, for which there are substantial body stores.

- **Thiamine deficiency** can develop quickly (within 3 weeks), and leads to Wernicke's encephalopathy. People with alcohol problems are particularly predisposed, but so are patients with prolonged (> 3 weeks) vomiting

- **Folate** stores are relatively small and deficiency can occur quickly, causing a macrocytic anaemia
- **Vitamin C deficiency** (scurvy) is much commoner than realized, and impairs wound healing. If prolonged, classic scurvy may occur, with the development of unusual 'corkscrew-shaped' hair, haemorrhages around the hair follicle, swollen spongy gums leading to loose teeth, spontaneous bruising and bleeding. Anaemia, which is usually hypochromic but can be normochromic also occurs. Vitamin C levels can be measured in the plasma, and also in the leukocyte– platelet layer of centrifuged blood – the 'buffy' layer. Treatment is with ascorbic acid
- **Iron** (microcytic anaemia, glossitis, cheilosis, koilonychia), **calcium** (proximal myopathy, perioral paraesthesia, tetany) and **magnesium** (myopathy not responding to calcium) deficiency can all occur in hospitalized patients

Nutritional support
Indications

In patients considered to be malnourished, consideration should always be given to nutritional support (Fig. 26.1).

Table 26.1 Feature of water-soluble vitamin deficiency

	Vitamin B$_1$	Vitamin B$_2$	Niacin	Vitamin B$_6$
Solubility	Water			
Common name	Thiamine	Riboflavin		Pyridoxine
Occurrence	• Cereals • Beans • Nuts • Pork, duck	• Dairy products • Offal • Leafy vegetables	• Plants • Meat • Fish	Found widely in plant and animal derived foods
Function	Essential cofactor in many enzyme systems, especially involving carbohydrate metabolism		Hydrogen acceptor in many oxidative reactions	Cofactor in metabolism of many amino acids
Cause of deficiency	• Dietary deficiency, e.g. milled rice • Alcoholism (usually due to dietary deficiency) • Prolonged vomiting, e.g. hyperemesis gravidarum, cancer especially with chemotherapy	Low dietary intake	Lost during the milling process of cereals – unless replaced deficiency occurs in those with cereal-only diet • Isoniazid therapy • Malabsorption syndromes (rare) • Carcinoid syndrome	• Dietary deficiency is very rare • Drugs can produce deficiency (e.g. isoniazid hydralazine penicillamine)
Consequence of deficiency	• 'Dry' beriberi; polyneuropathy, ± cerebral involvement with Wernicke–Korsakoff syndrome (causing dementia, ataxia, external ophthalmoplegia, nystagmus) • 'Wet' beriberi: oedema of the legs →ascites, pleural effusions (largely due to cardiac failure) • Vasodilatation (due to lactic acid) →bounding pulse	Clinical deficiency very rare: • Angular stomatitis • Red inflamed tongue • Seborrhoeic dermatitis • Conjunctivitis	Pellagra (→the 3 Ds): • **Dermatitis:** in sun-exposed areas of the skin →thickening, dry, hyperpigmentation • **Diarrhoea:** other GI symptoms include a red raw tongue, glossitis, angular stomatitis • **Dementia:** in severe cases, in milder cases, depression, apathy ad thought disorders	• Polyneuropathy • Rarely, some sideroblastic anaemias respond to B$_6$ • Some premenstrual tension symptoms may respond to B$_6$ supplementation
Diagnosis	• Clinical response to thiamine • Red cell (transketolase) before and after added thiamine		Clinical features	Clinical features
General treatment	Most vitamin deficiencies are not isolated, and accordingly multiple different vitamin supplements should be given, along with protein and calories			
Treatment	Supplemental thiamine – if due to ethyl alcohol abuse, thiamine must be given prior to carbohydrates	Riboflavin supplementation	Niacin supplementation	Vitamin B$_6$
Excess	Ataxia	No data		

Therapeutic diets

Many diets are useful for the treatment of specific gastrointestinal (GI) conditions and for non-specific symptoms (Table 26.2). Low protein diets tend not to be advised nowadays for either renal failure or hepatic encephalopathy.

Certain medical conditions will only improve or enable the patient to lead a normal life if they have a significant and long-term alteration to their diet. The use of a dietician is essential in these cases and you will also have to engage the patient in understanding the lifestyle modifications they will have to make to ensure their success. This can involve not only the patient but also the family and carer. Longer term follow up is essential but much of this can be passed onto the community services, outlining the diagnosis, treatment and exactly what the patient has been told or understands.

Table 26.2 Indications for specific diets

Diet	Indication	Principle
Gluten free	Coeliac disease	Total gluten withdrawal
Low lactose	Hypolactasia	Low in dairy products
High fibre	Constipation/ diverticular change	High content of insoluble fibre (e.g. bran)
Low residue	Subacute small bowel obstruction (e.g. Crohn's disease)	Low in fibre to reduce obstructive symptoms
Exclusion	Intractable irritable bowel	Bland diet for control of irritable bowel symptoms
Low salt	Cirrhosis, heart failure	Useful adjunct to diuretics in control of oedema and/or ascites
Elemental/ peptide	Crohn's disease	Liquid diet with nitrogen as either short peptides or amino acids

TOP TIPS

- Always consider the nutritional status of the patient
- Take a dietary history
- Enquire about weight loss or gain
- Refer to a dietician
- Engage the carers in any change to diet or lifestyle
- Ensure good communication with primary care on discharge

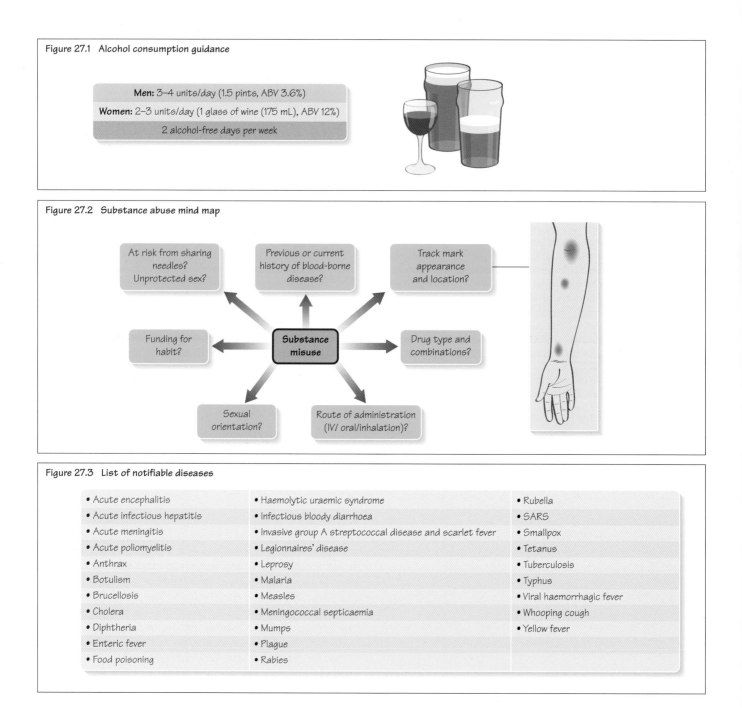

Figure 27.1 Alcohol consumption guidance

Men: 3–4 units/day (1.5 pints, ABV 3.6%)

Women: 2–3 units/day (1 glass of wine (175 mL), ABV 12%)

2 alcohol-free days per week

Figure 27.2 Substance abuse mind map

At risk from sharing needles? Unprotected sex?

Previous or current history of blood-borne disease?

Track mark appearance and location?

Funding for habit?

Substance misuse

Drug type and combinations?

Sexual orientation?

Route of administration (IV/ oral/inhalation)?

Figure 27.3 List of notifiable diseases

- Acute encephalitis
- Acute infectious hepatitis
- Acute meningitis
- Acute poliomyelitis
- Anthrax
- Botulism
- Brucellosis
- Cholera
- Diphtheria
- Enteric fever
- Food poisoning

- Haemolytic uraemic syndrome
- Infectious bloody diarrhoea
- Invasive group A streptococcal disease and scarlet fever
- Legionnaires' disease
- Leprosy
- Malaria
- Measles
- Meningococcal septicaemia
- Mumps
- Plague
- Rabies

- Rubella
- SARS
- Smallpox
- Tetanus
- Tuberculosis
- Typhus
- Viral haemorrhagic fever
- Whooping cough
- Yellow fever

This chapter covers the major factors that affect the health of the population – as a doctor you have a responsibility to look at the wider health agenda. There is an increasing focus on health promotion and educating the public to prevent disease and promote their own health. It is therefore essential that you acquire the knowledge and skills to help you educate patients effectively. You should use every opportunity to consider the patient as a whole and not just focus on the presenting complaint. Patients' lifestyles can have a profound effect not only on their presenting illnesses but how effective treatment will be and whether they can expect to make a full recovery. Consider the following:

- Alcohol
- Smoking
- Drugs
- Diet
- Nutrition

Alcohol

You will routinely take a full history from the patient including all of the above domains. However, how often will you use the information to better inform the patient?

- Do you advise on appropriate weekly alcohol consumption?
- Do you advise women of child-bearing age about the effects of alcohol on the unborn child?
- Do you know if the patient's alcohol consumption is having an effect on their family or work?
- If the patient asked for help whom would you refer them to?

The patient may widely underestimate the amount of alcohol they consume (Fig. 27.1) and you may have to rely on liver function tests to alert you to the problem. You may also get a more accurate history from relatives. Explaining to the patient the effect of their alcohol consumption on their presenting complaint or its effect on their long-term health is an opportunity not to be missed.

Smoking

It is very difficult for the patient to disguise the fact that they smoke and they usually give an accurate estimate of the number of cigarettes they consume. Whether their presenting complaint is related to their consumption or not, it is important to use time in the consultation to inform them of the help they can get to quit.

- What strategies do you know to help them quit?
- What support is available and how will they be followed up?
- Do others in the family smoke? Relapse rates are high in smokers who come from homes where other people also smoke, so lifestyle considerations are paramount

Drugs

Substance abuse and misuse is an increasingly common problem, with major implications for the patients' and families' health and psychosocial well being. You may not feel best equipped to deal with the issue but you might well be the first person in a health setting to recognize that the patient has a drug problem. Again, a full history from the patient and relatives or friends should reveal the extent of the problem. Discussion with the patient will reveal whether they are actively looking for support or indeed whether they do not want any medical interference in their habit. It is still essential that you have the discussion with the patient and are aware of how to refer them for further help. Documentation in the notes is also essential, as is the risk of blood-borne infections, when additional precautions are required by all health workers. You will need to document all the items shown in Fig. 27.2.

Diet and nutrition

Being overweight is a risk factor for many diseases like diabetes, cardiovascular disease and musculoskeletal disease and therefore plays a large part in the treatment plan for the patient. Telling them to lose weight is, however, unlikely to bring a positive result. The patient needs to understand the impact their weight has on their presenting complaint and their future morbidity. Enlist the help of relatives to discuss the lifestyle issues surrounding their weight and of course make a referral to a dietician.

Undernourishment is just as important and there are many reports of patients who are malnourished while in the hospital setting. Consider the following:

- Can the patient communicate their needs?
- Are they able to feed themselves?
- Do they have specific dietary requirements?
- Does their ethnicity impact on their eating (e.g. religious fasting)?
- Is the food presented appetizing?
- Does their medical condition make eating difficult (e.g. stroke)?

Alerting the team to potential malnourishment is important because it is likely to delay discharge and can add to the complications of the presenting medical condition.

Wider public health issues

The foundation curriculum also includes the need to have a wider understanding of public health issues. You should, therefore, not only consider the health of the patient in front of you but also consider the population risk factors for health:

- Genetics
- Social deprivation
- Health outcome inequalities amongst ethic minority communities
- Sexual behaviour and sexually transmitted diseases
- Occupation and unemployment
- Postcode health lottery
- Accidents

These are all issues within the curriculum that you need to be familiar with, and you will need to demonstrate knowledge in the following areas:

- Epidemiology and screening
- Data collection methods and their limitations
- Demographic data collection using ethnicity data to inform health promotion and care planning
- Conditions that are notifiable and how to inform the relevant competent authority (Fig. 27.3)

The emphasis on health promotion and public health is important for all doctors to learn and understand. While it may seem less glamorous than interventional medicine it is important for the long-term health of the patient, the community and the country.

TOP TIPS

- Take a full history of health-related lifestyle issues
- Think about health advice to all patients
- Discuss consumption of alcohol and drugs
- Offer further expert guidance from other members of team

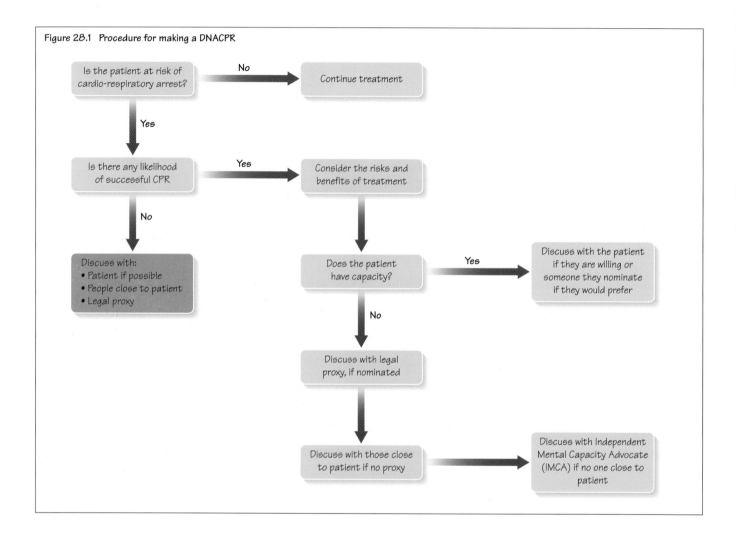

Figure 28.1 Procedure for making a DNACPR

Is the patient at risk of cardio-respiratory arrest? → **No** → Continue treatment

↓ **Yes**

Is there any likelihood of successful CPR → **Yes** → Consider the risks and benefits of treatment

↓ **No**

Discuss with:
• Patient if possible
• People close to patient
• Legal proxy

Consider the risks and benefits of treatment ↓

Does the patient have capacity? → **Yes** → Discuss with the patient if they are willing or someone they nominate if they would prefer

↓ **No**

Discuss with legal proxy, if nominated

↓

Discuss with those close to patient if no proxy → Discuss with Independent Mental Capacity Advocate (IMCA) if no one close to patient

This chapter covers the issues that doctors face when assessing the risk–benefit analysis of decisions to treat patients, specifically whether or not to perform cardiopulmonary resuscitation (CPR). Such decisions must be made in the patient's best overall interests.

There are a number of important issues to be considered when making a DNACPR (do not attempt CPR decision).

Ethical and legal considerations

The Human Rights Act 1998 and Articles of the European Convention on Human Rights dictate that decisions about resuscitation status must consider the views of the patient and their relatives.

In 2010 the GMC published the online *Treatment and Care Towards the End of Life* which clearly sets out a doctor's duties and responsibilities for all aspects of end of life care, including decisions about resuscitation (see www.gmc-uk.org/guidance/ethical_guidance/end_of_life_care.asp).

Where patients have capacity to decide, they may chose not to undergo CPR; where patients lack capacity, legally, decisions need to be based on whether treatment is in a patient's 'best interests' (in England, Wales and Northern Ireland) or 'benefits' a patient (in Scotland) as set out in the Mental Capacity Act 2005 and Adults with Incapacity (Scotland) Act 2000.

When to consider making a DNACPR decision

Where death is imminent and CPR will not be effective, then making and recording a decision not to attempt CPR in advance will allow the patient to die in a peaceful and dignified manner. Leaving this decision until the time of arrest may lead to inappropriate or unwanted CPR and deny the patient the choice of deciding where they wish to die.

Even when CPR may be effective at restarting the heart, it may not be clinically appropriate or wanted by the patient. The decision to attempt CPR or not must consider the values and beliefs of the patient. This information must be gathered from the patient (if possible) or from those who know the patient best – either relatives or a person with appropriate legal proxy to make such decisions.

Where no such person exists, the Mental Capacity Act 2005 requires doctors in England and Wales to discuss such decisions with an Independent Mental Capacity Advocate (IMCA).

Discussions about CPR

If a patient is thought to be at risk of cardiorespiratory arrest and the healthcare team feel that CPR will not be successful, you must consider whether it is appropriate to tell the patient about this decision. If the decision is made not to discuss this with the patient, then you should seek their consent to share such information with those close to them. If they lack capacity, then this decision should be shared with a legal proxy if appointed and people close to the patient (Fig. 28.1).

In cases where you feel CPR may be effective, you must weigh the benefits of prolonging life against the burdens and risks to the patient. 'Best interests' is not a medical decision but a value judgement and needs to be based on the views of the patient, not the doctor. You should offer patients the opportunity to discuss their views and assuming they wish to have this discussion, provide them with relevant information to inform their views. However, you must not force them to have such a conversation.

What if a person lacks capacity?

As mentioned earlier, when a patient lacks capacity, you should discuss it with a legal proxy if such person exists. If not, then you should discuss it with the people closest to the patient. However, it is vital that you don't leave them thinking they are making a formal decision on the patient's behalf. This can leave them feeling guilty later on. When a patient lacks capacity, the decision is made by the medical staff, or occasionally a court, about what is in the patient's 'best interests'. The role of the family is to guide staff as to the patient's beliefs and wishes.

What if there is a disagreement?

If the patient wants to receive CPR, even though it is not felt to be clinically appropriate, you should make sure they have accurate information and explore the reasons behind their decision. It may be that a compromise can be reached, but if not, then in general, the patient's wishes should be respected. A doctor cannot be forced to provide a treatment that is not medically justified and should you decide to refuse, you must explain your reasons to the patient and explain their options, including a second opinion. You should probably also discuss it with your trust's legal department or defence union first. Similar obligations apply when dealing with the legal proxy for a patient.

When a patient lacks capacity and there is no legal proxy, even though relatives should not bear the burden of making a final decision, you should still aim to reach a consensus. Where disagreement arises, either within the healthcare team or with relatives, options include involving an advocate, seeking a second opinion or holding a case conference. If despite this, there is still disagreement, it would again be advisable to seek legal advice.

Practical Issues

All trusts are required to have a DNACPR policy. It is worth making yourself familiar with this. It will set out who can make DNACPR decisions and how to document them. These decisions need to be made by an experienced, senior clinician. There may also be a form to record such decisions. This will document who made the decision, when, why and with whom it was discussed and may also specify a review date. Once made, the decision should be clearly recorded and communicated to all relevant healthcare professionals, whilst still respecting the patient's privacy.

TOP TIPS

DNACPR decisions:
- Need to be made by a senior clinician, clearly documented and relevant healthcare workers informed
- Should be discussed with the patient, family and legal proxies as appropriate
- Must be made on the basis of 'best interests' or 'benefits'
- Should be reached by consensus if at all possible
- Are not the same as withdrawing treatment

Figure 29.1 The causes and treatment of pain in palliative care

(a) Causes of pain in cancer patients

(b) Analgesic ladder

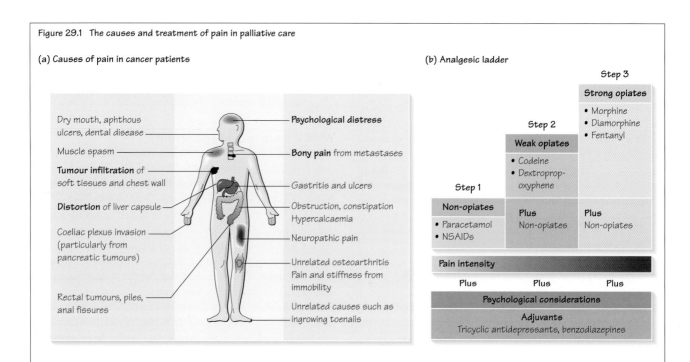

(c) Treatment for different types of pain

Cause of pain	Opioid sensitivity	Primary treatment	Examples of other options
Large infiltrating tumour mass	Partial	• Opioids • NSAIDs • Steroids	• Treat tumour bulk, e.g. radiotherapy
Musculoskeletal pain	Insensitive	• Peripherally acting analgesics (paracetamol, NSAIDs) • Physiotherapy • Massage	• Benzodiazepines
Colic	Insensitive	• Treat underlying cause, e.g. constipation • Anticholinergics	• In bowel obstruction consider reversal, e.g. with surgery or anticancer therapy. Steroids and/or octreotide if reversal is not possible
Bone pain	Partial	• NSAIDs • Opioids	• Radiotherapy • Orthopaedic surgery – especially if a metastasis has caused an unstable joint or long bone at risk of fracture • Bisphosphonates
Capsular stretching, e.g. liver capsule pain	Partial	• NSAIDs • Opioids • Steroids	• Chemotherapy
Nerve pain – symptoms include pain that is described as burning, stabbing or shooting in nature and there may be altered sensation	Partial (?)	• Tricyclic antidepressants • Antiepileptics (Gabapentin) • Opioids	• Steroids • Nerve blocks • Radiotherapy
NSAIDs (non-steroidal anti-inflammatory drugs)			

Palliative care is an approach that improves the quality of life of patients and their families facing the problems associated with life-threatening illness, through the prevention and relief of suffering by means of early identification and impeccable assessment and treatment of pain and other problems, physical, psychosocial and spiritual. (World Health Organization definition)

There is a perception that palliation should be reserved for patients who are imminently dying. Palliative care is appropriate for any advanced progressive malignant and non-malignant illness. All clinicians need skills in palliative management; however some patients, particularly those with complex needs, need referral to a specialist palliative care service. This chapter covers the two symptom control issues of pain management and the dying process.

Pain

Assessment

A proper pain assessment is the cornerstone of effectively alleviating symptoms. Pain in progressive illness is complex and focusing exclusively on the physical causes explains why pain relief may be inadequate. When assessing the physical cause, consider that pain may relate to the cancer, e.g. local infiltration (visceral, nerve and bone pain), to disabilities relating to chronic illness (e.g. musculoskeletal problems) or to co-morbidities (Fig. 29.1a). Consequently there are often many causes and sites of pain and each must be assessed by taking a careful history, noting:

- Where the pain is, and radiates to
- Type and severity of pain
- The onset of pain
- Response to analgesics
- Exacerbating and alleviating factors

Physical examination often establishes the diagnosis, though it may be necessary to perform investigations such as X rays, isotope bone scans, computed tomography scans, etc.

A complete assessment includes an appraisal of:

- **Emotional pain**: when faced with advanced illness, patients frequently experience depression, uncertainty, despair, anger and fear
- **Social pain**: socially isolated patients can feel unsafe, and those who are financially insecure can feel threatened

Treatment (Fig. 29.1c)

Analgesics

The World Health Organization advocates a three-step ladder for prescribing analgesics (Fig. 29.1b). Analgesics should be prescribed regularly. Inadequate pain control at one step requires a move to the next step. Adjuvant co-analgesics can be used at each step for treating that element of the pain which is opioid insensitive.

Opioids

The correct use of opioids has made a major impact on the management of pain in patients with advanced disease. Unfortunately unfounded fears by professionals and patients about the use of strong opioids, lack of understanding about how opioids should be prescribed and an inability to recognize pain that is opioid resistant can lead to ineffective prescribing.

Prescribing opioids Morphine continues to be the 'gold standard' analgesic. Oral morphine is available in two forms: immediate acting (4-hourly) and slow release (12- and 24-hourly) preparations. When prescribed correctly it is a safe, predictable and reliable drug. Correct prescribing of morphine requires that:

- Morphine should be given orally unless this is impossible
- It must be prescribed regularly to pre-empt pain
- In acute pain, rapid titration of the dose is best achieved using regular immediate-release opioid
- Extra doses for breakthrough and incident pain must be co-prescribed and used as necessary
- Side effects, particularly constipation, should be anticipated and prevented
- Pain should be continuously reassessed

Failure of opioid therapy may be due to incorrect prescription, poor compliance or the pain being opioid insensitive.

Side effects of morphine
- Constipation is virtually universal; a laxative should always be co-prescribed
- Nausea and vomiting (less common)
- Drowsiness in 50% of patients; this wears off after a week on a stable dose. Explanation and reassurance are usually all that is necessary
- Other side effects include confusion, sweating, dry mouth, itch, hallucinations and myoclonus

Alternative opioids Morphine metabolites can be responsible for side effects, and morphine is dependent on the kidney for excretion. Alternative opioids, e.g. fentanyl (transdermal preparation) and oxycodone, may be used when opioid-sensitive pain exists but morphine is causing excessive side effects or is contraindicated.

Terminal phase of illness

Healthcare professionals should ensure that the dying patient has a 'good death'. Physical symptoms, including pain, must be controlled and wider issues (e.g. the needs of the family) should be appreciated. Anticipating symptoms and good communication with relatives is fundamental; patient pathways such as the 'Liverpool Care Pathway' enable optimal management. The three commonest symptoms are:

- **Pain**: where possible ask about pain and check for easily reversible causes. Some patients may need to start opioids, and those on regular opioids, who cannot take oral medication, will need parenteral (often subcutaneous) therapy
- **Noisy, moist breathing**: when a patient's condition deteriorates there are likely to be changes in respiration that can be predicted. Often the pattern of breathing alters and it is reassuring to the relatives to be warned of these potential changes. As the patient weakens, the ability to cough up secretions is lost. It can usually be relieved by anticholinergic drugs
- **Restlessness and distress**: terminal distress, preterminal agitation, terminal restlessness and terminal anguish are all terms used to describe agitation and distress in patients close to death. Terminal restlessness reflects significant suffering on the part of the patient and causes considerable distress to the relatives who witness it. It is particularly important to assess the patient and rule out easily reversible causes, e.g. catheterization for urinary retention. Sedation should be offered to ease a patient's distress and midazolam is often the drug of choice

TOP TIPS
- Treat the whole patient
- Be aware of side effects of medication
- Review medication and dosage regularly
- Explain to the patient and carers what you are prescribing
- Enquire about new symptoms daily

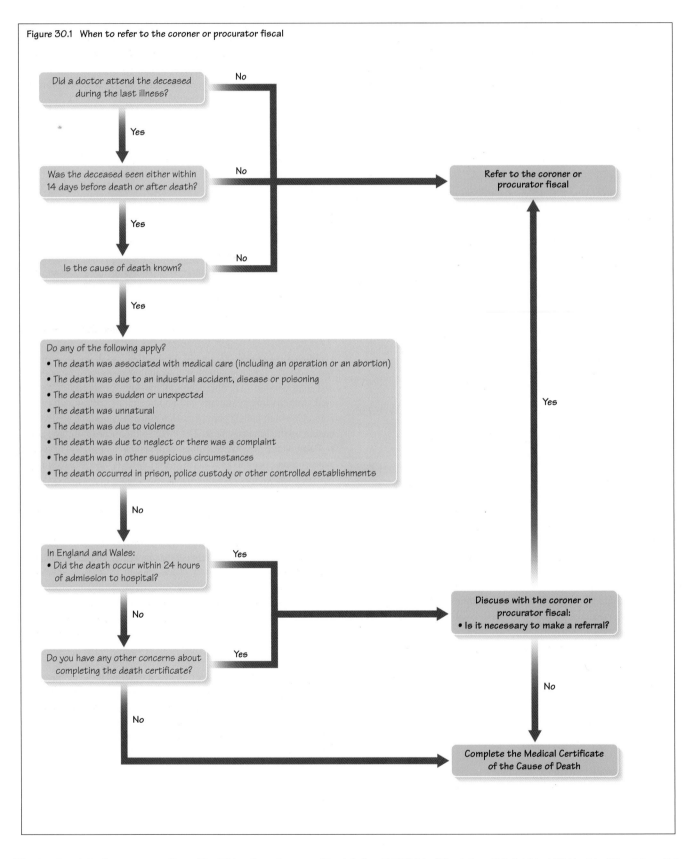

Figure 30.1 When to refer to the coroner or procurator fiscal

Did a doctor attend the deceased during the last illness?

No

Yes

Was the deceased seen either within 14 days before death or after death?

No

Refer to the coroner or procurator fiscal

Yes

Is the cause of death known?

No

Yes

Do any of the following apply?
• The death was associated with medical care (including an operation or an abortion)
• The death was due to an industrial accident, disease or poisoning
• The death was sudden or unexpected
• The death was unnatural
• The death was due to violence
• The death was due to neglect or there was a complaint
• The death was in other suspicious circumstances
• The death occurred in prison, police custody or other controlled establishments

Yes

No

In England and Wales:
• Did the death occur within 24 hours of admission to hospital?

Yes

No

Discuss with the coroner or procurator fiscal:
• Is it necessary to make a referral?

Do you have any other concerns about completing the death certificate?

Yes

No

No

Complete the Medical Certificate of the Cause of Death

This chapter covers how and when to complete a Medical Certificate of the Cause of Death (MCCD). In addition, it covers when you should refer the death to the coroner (in England, Wales and Northern Ireland) or to the procurator fiscal (in Scotland).

As a doctor you will be called upon to complete a MCCD. You should only complete a MCCD if you were involved in caring for the deceased during the final illness and know the cause of death.

The MCCD is a permanent legal record of the fact of death. It permits the formal registration of death and the issuing of a death certificate, which allows the family to arrange a funeral and to settle the deceased's estate. It also provides important information about the causes of death that will be used for epidemiological purposes.

How to complete a MCCD

The MCCD is set out in two parts (I and II). Part I is used to show the immediate cause of death and any underlying cause or causes. You should only use Part II if there was any significant condition or disease that contributed to the death but was not part of the sequence that led directly to the patient's death.

When completing Part I, you should start with the immediate and direct cause of death. On each line below, you should go back through the sequence of events or conditions that led to the death. The condition on the lowest line of Part I should have caused all of the conditions above it. Most routine mortality statistics are based on what is on the bottom line, i.e. the underlying cause.

For example:

I (a) *Disease or condition leading directly to death* – Bronchopneumonia

I (b) *Other disease or condition, if any, leading to* I (a) – *Intracerebral haemorrhage*

I (c) *Other disease or condition, if any, leading to* I (b) – *Cerebral metastases*

I (d) *Other disease or condition, if any, leading to* I (c) – *Squamous cell carcinoma of left main bronchus*

You should list in Part II any other conditions that contributed to the patient's death but were not part of the main sequence leading to death. However, you are not required to list all the conditions present at death in Part II. In the example above, the person may have died sooner because they also had diabetes mellitus. In some cases, a single disease may be wholly responsible.

Remember, you must write out the cause of death in full. 'Cerebrovascular accident' is acceptable but 'CVA' is not.

A common mistake when completing a MCCD is to confuse the cause of death with the mode of death. For example, 'cardiac arrest' describes how death occurred and not the cause of death. Other unacceptable terms on the MCCD include:
- Asphyxia
- Respiratory arrest
- Exhaustion
- Shock
- Heart failure

Finally, you must sign the certificate, print your name and add your qualifications, address and the date. If the death occurred in hospital, the name of the consultant who was responsible for the care of the patient must also be given.

When to inform the coroner or procurator fiscal

The coroner, or procurator fiscal in Scotland, is responsible for investigating violent or unnatural deaths, sudden deaths of unknown cause and deaths that occurred in prison, police custody or other controlled establishments. A decision tree is given in Fig. 30.1.

The underlying principle is: if you have any doubt about whether to refer, contact the coroner or procurator fiscal.

What does the coroner or procurator fiscal need to know?

When referring a death to the coroner or procurator fiscal, you should include the following information:
- Name of deceased
- Age and/or date of birth
- Home address
- Religion/ethnic origin
- Place, date and time of death
- Nearest relatives (if known) and whether they have any special needs, e.g. translation needed
- General practitioner (if known)
- History
- Cause of death, if ascertained, and whether the death can be certified
- The name of the doctor who proposes to sign any death certificate
- Whether the family have any concerns about the circumstances of the death

What happens next?

Following discussion or initial inquiries, the coroner or procurator fiscal may determine that no further action is needed. This is likely to be the decision if the doctor reporting the death is prepared to issue a MCCD and if the death occurred from natural causes and does not require further investigation.

However, the coroner or procurator fiscal may require further investigations. This could include a postmortem.

In England and Wales, further investigations will typically be undertaken by the coroner's officers. If the cause of death is still unclear after the postmortem, the coroner must hold an inquest. In Scotland, the procurator fiscal may request a police report.

The hospital may request a postmortem even if the coroner or procurator fiscal decides that the death does not require any further action. If this is the case, the deceased's relatives must give consent for the postmortem.

TOP TIPS

- If you have any doubts about completing the death certificate, you should discuss these with the coroner or procurator fiscal
- The MCCD asks for the cause of death and not the mode of death
- Print your name under your signature

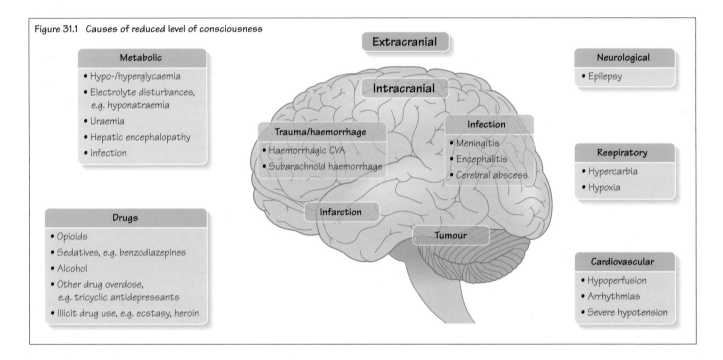

Figure 31.1 Causes of reduced level of consciousness

Extracranial

Metabolic
- Hypo-/hyperglycaemia
- Electrolyte disturbances, e.g. hyponatraemia
- Uraemia
- Hepatic encephalopathy
- Infection

Intracranial

Trauma/haemorrhage
- Haemorrhagic CVA
- Subarachnoid haemorrhage

Infection
- Meningitis
- Encephalitis
- Cerebral abscess

Infarction

Tumour

Drugs
- Opioids
- Sedatives, e.g. benzodiazepines
- Alcohol
- Other drug overdose, e.g. tricyclic antidepressants
- Illicit drug use, e.g. ecstasy, heroin

Neurological
- Epilepsy

Respiratory
- Hypercarbia
- Hypoxia

Cardiovascular
- Hypoperfusion
- Arrhythmias
- Severe hypotension

This chapter covers:
- History and examination of the unconscious patient
- ABCDE of assessment
- Investigations and treatment
- When to call for help

Patients may present as new admissions with decreased levels of consciousness or may deteriorate whilst an inpatient. It is important to have a method of assessment for any such patient. They may present with life-threatening conditions or have life-threatening complications requiring immediate management. A logical approach to assessing these patients improves safety, makes sure that nothing is overlooked and also reduces doctor anxiety.

History

The patient is unlikely to be able to give any history but this can be sought from other sources – family, bystanders, paramedics, GP and hospital staff.

Review the patient's notes and drug charts for indications of possible causes (Fig. 31.1).

Review the ambulance notes, these often give a good indication of initial method of presentation.

Important points in the history include:
- History of head injury? **This may indicate a possible intracranial haemorrhage needing urgent management**
- Any previous similar episodes?
- Any previous neurological symptoms or headaches? **A patient that complains of a sudden severe headache may have a subarachnoid haemorrhage**
- Are they known epileptic?

- Are they diabetic?
- Are they on any medication? Is there any possibility of overdose? **Important medications include opioids and sedative medications such as benzodiazepines**
- Any other past medical history
- Any history of arrhythmias/palpitations? **A history of atrial fibrillation would raise the suspicion of a cerebrovascular accident (CVA)**
- Any possible illicit drug use?

Examination

Examination and initial treatment may occur simultaneously. As with any unwell patient, your approach should be ABCDE. Important aspects in the unconscious patients are as follows.

Airway

Is the airway patent? Are there any signs of obstruction? Signs of obstruction may include snoring/gurgling or paradoxical chest movements. If the airway is not patent or there are signs of obstruction **senior help should be sought**. Anaesthetic assistance may be required.

Are they at risk of aspiration (see explanation in D-Disability)?

If necessary, provide airway support with a chin lift/jaw thrust and insert an oropharyngeal airway. NB a jaw thrust rather than a chin lift/head tilt should be used in patients with suspected cervical spine trauma. Give oxygen at 15 L/min via non-rebreathing mask.

Breathing

Auscultate the chest. Are respiratory efforts adequate (good respiratory rate, depth of respiration, SPO_2)? May require support or intubation and ventilation if not adequate. **Call for senior help and an anaesthetist.**

Circulation

Check blood pressure and pulse. Inadequate circulation may be a cause of a reduced level of consciousness. Hypertension with bradycardia may be a sign of raised intracranial pressure (Cushing's reflex). It is important to maintain an adequate circulation, and fluid boluses may be initially helpful. Insert an IV cannula and start IV fluids.

Disability

The Glasgow Coma Score (GCS) is often used to assess the level of consciousness. This is a score out of 15 and is made up of three elements: eye opening, verbal and motor responses.

Assessing GCS score can sometimes be difficult. A simpler method of assessment is the AVPU score, which relates to the response level of the patient; are they:

- **A**lert (A)?
- Responsive to **V**oice (V)?
- Responsive to **P**ain only (P)?
- **U**nresponsive (U)?

An AVPU score of P or lower tends to correlate with a GCS or 8 or less. A GCS of 8 or less or an AVPU score of P or U should alert you to possible airway compromise – the patient is unable to protect their own airway and may be at risk of aspiration. **Senior help and anaesthetic assistance should be sought**.

Pupillary response – are the pupils equal and responsive to light? Unequal or unreactive pupils may indicate an intracranial cause (Fig. 31.1). Pinpoint pupils may indicate opioid overdose. Large pupils could indicate tricyclic antidepressant overdose.

Don't ever forget glucose – remember to check a blood glucose level; hypoglycaemia is an easily treatable cause of reduced level of consciousness.

Examination/Everything Else

A full systems examination should be undertaken, including a full neurological examination to assess for any localizing signs.

Investigations

Specific investigations are essential and will help diagnosis.

1 Blood tests:
  - FBC – a raised white cell count may be a sign of an infective cause
  - U&E – ?electrolyte abnormalities or acute renal failure with uraemia
  - LFT – deranged liver function tests may raise suspicion of possible hepatic encephalopathy but may be deranged for many other causes. If suspicion is high an ammonia level should be checked
  - Glucose – high or low glucose may be a possible cause
  - Arterial blood gas (ABG) – ?hypoxia, hypercarbia or severe acidosis
2 ECG – assess for arrhythmias.
3 Compute tomography (CT) head – assess for intracranial pathology (haemorrhage, tumour, infection).
4 Lumbar puncture – may be indicated if meningitis or encephalitis is suspected, though usually a CT head is performed first.

Management

Management of the unconscious patient is largely supportive whilst a diagnosis is sought. The generic management described above is focused on providing airway support, oxygenation and maintaining a good blood pressure/circulation.

In addition more specific management may include:
- Naloxone – if opioid overdose is suspected
- Treatment of hypoglycaemia
- Intracranial lesions/haemorrhage will need discussion with a neurosurgeon

TOP TIPS

- ABCDE
- Call for senior help
- Call for anaesthetist if AVPU score is P or U
- Give oxygen and fluids
- Check the glucose

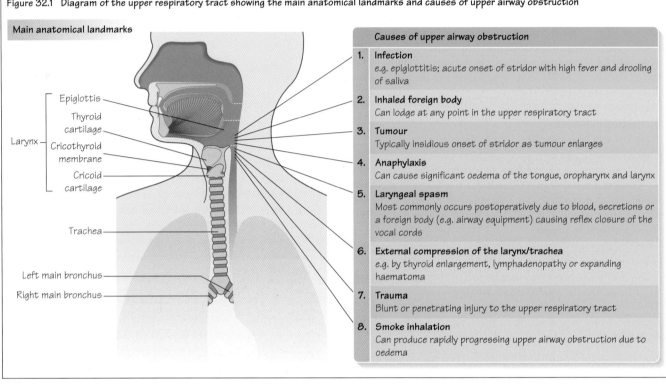

Figure 32.1 Diagram of the upper respiratory tract showing the main anatomical landmarks and causes of upper airway obstruction

This chapter covers:
- Aetiology of stridor
- Taking a history and making the diagnosis
- Management of stridor and calling for help

What is stridor?

Stridor is a distinctive harsh sound heard during breathing when there is a partial obstruction in the upper part of the airway. The obstruction causes turbulence in the flow of air in the airway and it is this turbulent flow that is heard as stridor. The presence of stridor implies that the patient has a significant airway obstruction but it is important to recognize that the loudness of the stridor does not equate with the severity of the obstruction. Depending on its aetiology, stridor can develop progressively over several days or weeks or can present very acutely.

Use the ABC approach to assessing and managing the patient. Airway problems can be rapidly life threatening and must be recognized and treated very quickly. If you are worried about a patient's airway it is essential to ask for senior help immediately.

What you see

The exact presentation of a patient with stridor will depend on the cause of their airway problem (Fig. 32.1). The patient is likely to be in the position in which they find it easiest to breathe, often sitting up very straight. **DO NOT LIE THE PATIENT DOWN FLAT OR RECLINE THEM.** They are likely to show signs of respiratory distress such as tachypnoea and use of accessory muscles. Their oxygen saturations may be low. The patient is likely to be very frightened and there may be cardiovascular signs such as tachycardia and hypertension due to stimulation of the sympathetic nervous system. If the upper airway obstruction is due to an infective cause, the patient may have a fever and be reluctant to swallow due to pain. If they can't swallow they will be dribbling.

History

Obtaining the history is important but due to their airway compromise and breathing difficulties the patient may not be able to provide you with any information. A relative, friend or paramedic may be able to provide useful information about the events leading up to admission. In your history important features to investigate include any previous history of upper airway problems or surgery, symptoms such as a fever or sore throat, any history of direct trauma to the throat or neck or a history of severe allergic reactions. Your history should also establish the duration over which symptoms have developed as well as determining past medical history, drug history and allergies.

Management

The priorities in managing a patient with stridor are
- Get help rapidly from an anaesthetist and ENT specialist and your experienced senior colleagues
- Avoid any actions that will worsen the airway obstruction
- The patient should be left in the position in which they are most comfortable

- Give high-flow oxygen through a non-rebreathing mask as soon as the airway problem is recognized
- Continuous monitoring of vital signs with pulse oximeter, blood pressure cuff and ECG
- Your examination of the patient should disturb them as little as possible. **DO NOT ATTEMPT TO LOOK IN THE MOUTH AND DO NOT PUT ANY INSTRUMENTS IN THE MOUTH** – this can distress the patient and make the situation worse
- Wait for the anaesthetist to arrive and they will examine the airway
- Most investigations can be deferred until the airway is secured after which time a full set of blood tests, arterial blood gases, chest X-ray and ECG can be carried out. In the majority of cases the results of these investigations will not influence your management sufficiently to justify carrying them out on a frightened patient
- A clear history of choking following foreign body inhalation is an **exception** to this and should be managed with back blows and abdominal thrusts

What to do while waiting for help to arrive

There are some treatments that may help a patient with partial airway obstruction until the specialist team arrives and the necessary arrangements are made.
- Nebulized adrenaline has the effect of reducing mucosal swelling in the airway, helping to limit the obstruction. It is simple to do – administer 1 mg via a nebulizer
- This is only a temporary measure and definitive treatment is still needed

Ongoing management

- Be alert for changes in the patient's condition. They can become exhausted or the obstruction can progress
- If a patient with airways obstruction becomes unconscious it is appropriate to use simple measures to support their airway. These include a jaw thrust or head tilt and chin lift
- Airway procedures such as the insertion of an oropharyngeal airway and bag–mask ventilation may be needed but should only be undertaken by an experienced person. At this stage help from an experienced anaesthetist is *vitally* important
- If the situation proceeds to cardiopulmonary arrest it should be managed according to the ALS algorithm

Dealing with a patient with an airway problem can be very stressful and early recognition and involvement of experienced senior colleagues is the key. Remember that the patient may be terrified and a calm, reassuring approach from their doctors and nurses will help enormously.

TOP TIPS
- Keep the patient with stridor sitting up
- Call for help
- Give oxygen and nebulized adrenaline
- Don't put instruments in the mouth
- Keep calm and reassure the patient

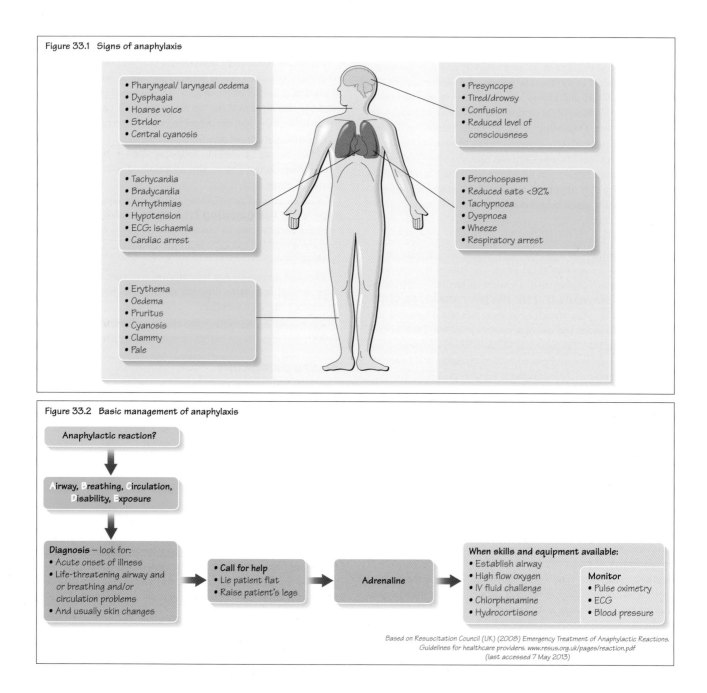

Figure 33.1 Signs of anaphylaxis

- Pharyngeal/ laryngeal oedema
- Dysphagia
- Hoarse voice
- Stridor
- Central cyanosis

- Presyncope
- Tired/drowsy
- Confusion
- Reduced level of consciousness

- Tachycardia
- Bradycardia
- Arrhythmias
- Hypotension
- ECG: ischaemia
- Cardiac arrest

- Bronchospasm
- Reduced sats <92%
- Tachypnoea
- Dyspnoea
- Wheeze
- Respiratory arrest

- Erythema
- Oedema
- Pruritus
- Cyanosis
- Clammy
- Pale

Figure 33.2 Basic management of anaphylaxis

Anaphylactic reaction?

Airway, Breathing, Circulation, Disability, Exposure

Diagnosis – look for:
- Acute onset of illness
- Life-threatening airway and or breathing and/or circulation problems
- And usually skin changes

- Call for help
- Lie patient flat
- Raise patient's legs

Adrenaline

When skills and equipment available:
- Establish airway
- High flow oxygen
- IV fluid challenge
- Chlorphenamine
- Hydrocortisone

Monitor
- Pulse oximetry
- ECG
- Blood pressure

Based on Resuscitation Council (UK) (2008) Emergency Treatment of Anaphylactic Reactions. Guidelines for healthcare providers. www.resus.org.uk/pages/reaction.pdf (last accessed 7 May 2013)

This chapter covers:
- What is anaphylaxis?
- Presentation and diagnosis
- Management

Anaphylaxis is a serious type I hypersensitivity reaction – a clinical syndrome, involving multiple organ systems, that is rapid in onset and may cause death. The term anaphylaxis now describes both 'anaphylactic' and 'anaphylactoid' reactions, with subdivision into allergic and non-allergic only after follow-up testing.

Incidence is underestimated at 175–1000 cases in the UK each year.

Mechanism

Susceptible individuals exposed to an allergen undergo a silent clinical episode, become sensitized and form IgE antibodies. Exposure to the allergen on a subsequent occasion triggers a cascade and release of biochemical mediators from mast cells and basophils. A very small amount of allergen is required to set off this reaction.

Non-allergic reactions activate mast cells directly.

Triggers

A plethora of triggers exist; the most common are food, drugs and venom. Nuts are the most commonly implicated food; penicillins are most frequently implicated antibiotics. Cross-reactivity with cephalosporins is approximately 8% and so should be avoided if there is a history of severe penicillin reaction. Contrast media is the most common cause of non-allergic anaphylaxis.

Presentation/range of symptoms

Clinical manifestations are the result of an immediate and sustained release of inflammatory mediators. The more rapidly that these events occur following allergen exposure, the more severe the reaction and the more critically unwell the patient is likely to be. This is related to the source and route of exposure:
- *IV bolus*: rapid onset, within minutes, likely cardiovascular system (CVS) collapse
- *Rectal*: 15–30 minutes (urticaria, angioedema or asthma are common)
- *Insect stings*: 10–15 minutes
- *Gelatin infusion*: 15–30 minutes
- *Latex allergy* (via peritoneum, mucosa or skin): > 30 minutes
- *Food*: 30–35 minutes

Intravenous drug administration results in a faster onset and is more commonly implicated. All healthcare professionals giving IV drugs must be competent to recognize and manage anaphylaxis.

What questions to ask the patient?

A focused history is essential – speedy diagnosis and expedient resuscitation will be needed to counter a rapidly deteriorating clinical condition. Important points are:
- *Past medical history*: bronchospasm is more severe in asthmatic patients, particularly if poorly controlled
- *Allergy*: latex allergy is more prevalent in patients who underwent surgery in the first year of life and in spina bifida. There is cross-reactivity between latex sensitivity and certain foods (bananas, chestnuts, avocado). Is there known anaphylaxis or exposure to a known allergen?
- *Exposure history*: new foods, medication and chemicals. Route of exposure

Examination/anything else to look for?

The initial diagnosis of anaphylaxis is presumptive. The degree of extremis is gauged largely from eliciting the spectrum of clinical signs using a systems-based approach, according to Advanced Life Support guidelines. Hypersensitivity reactions are graded from I to IV using a clinical severity scale.

I	Cutaneous–mucous signs: erythema, urticaria +/− angioedema
II	Moderate multivisceral signs: cutaneous–mucous signs +/− hypotension +/− tachycardia +/− dyspnoea +/− GIT disturbances
III	Life-threatening mono- or multivisceral signs Cardiovascular collapse, tachycardia (or bradycardia) +/− cardiac dysrhythmia +/− bronchospasm +/− cutaneous-mucous signs +/− GIT disturbances
IV	CARDIAC ARREST

The common clinical findings (Fig. 33.1) result largely from increased bronchial and gastrointestinal smooth muscle tone and capillary leakage. Cutaneous signs may be absent. Changes in vascular permeability can result in the transfer of 50% of the intravascular volume into the interstitial space **within 10 minutes**. A reflex protective mechanism, allowing the ventricles time to fill despite massive volume depletion, explains why a bradycardia can sometimes be present.

Practical management

Basic management follows the Resuscitation Council (UK) guidelines (Fig. 33.2):
1 Recognition of illness severity.
2 Call for senior help immediately.
3 Remove trigger (if possible).
4 Assessment and intervention based on ABCDE approach.
5 Give IV fluids and 100% oxygen.
6 Raise the legs if BP is low.
7 Give adrenaline IM if indicated (life-threatening features).
8 Adrenaline IV should only be given by those trained to do so.
9 Consider antihistamines and oral steroids for up to 3 days.
10 Referral to allergy specialist for follow up.
11 'Yellow card' anaphylaxis report (if drug reaction is suspected).
12 Consider prescription of auto-injector.

Use normal saline 0.9% or Hartmann's solution (**not** colloids) as the fluid for resuscitation.

Documentation, including event circumstances, timing of treatment administration and blood testing, is extremely important.

Patients should receive written documentation of the events, be given a MedicAlert bracelet and their GP informed.

Investigations

Early The only helpful diagnostic blood test required at the time of the reaction is serum tryptase. When released systemically it indicates anaphylaxis has occurred. Normal mast cell tryptase does not exclude anaphylaxis.

A 5–10 mL clotted blood sample should be taken:
- Initially as soon as resuscitation has commenced
- 1–2 hours after symptom onset
- (If this is missed take a timed sample within 6 hours)
- Take a third sample at 24 hours or at follow up (for baseline tryptase levels)

All samples must indicate time of collection and date.

Later Refer to a regional allergy centre to be fully investigated using IgE assays and skin tests.

TOP TIPS
- Anaphylaxis can happen to anyone at any time!
- High index of suspicion
- Call for help
- Give fluids, oxygen and adrenaline

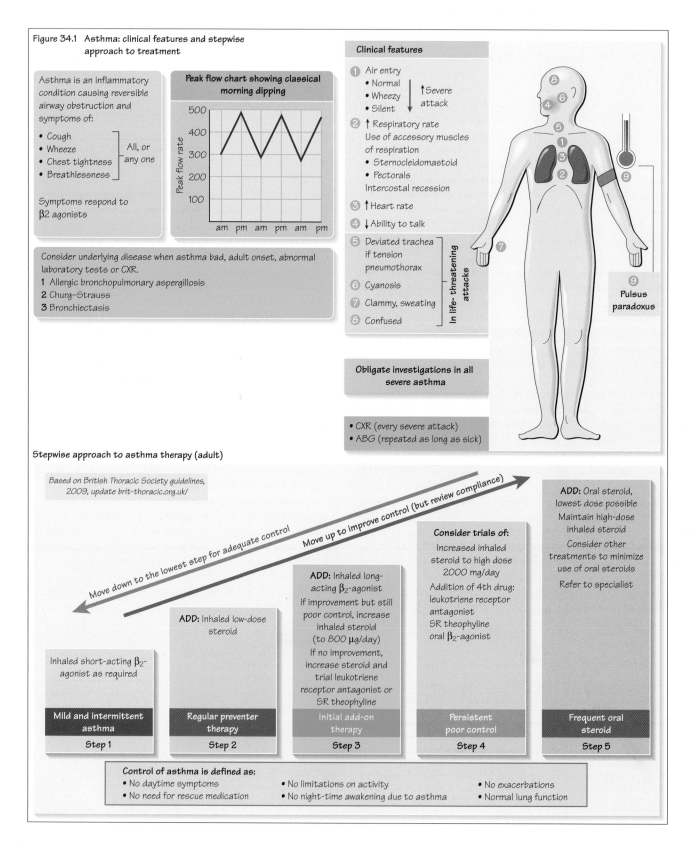

Figure 34.1 Asthma: clinical features and stepwise approach to treatment

Asthma is an inflammatory condition causing reversible airway obstruction and symptoms of:

- Cough
- Wheeze   } All, or
- Chest tightness   } any one
- Breathlessness

Symptoms respond to β2 agonists

Peak flow chart showing classical morning dipping

Consider underlying disease when asthma bad, adult onset, abnormal laboratory tests or CXR.
1 Allergic bronchopulmonary aspergillosis
2 Churg–Strauss
3 Bronchiectasis

Clinical features

1 Air entry
- Normal
- Wheezy   } ↑Severe attack
- Silent

2 ↑ Respiratory rate
Use of accessory muscles of respiration
- Sternocleidomastoid
- Pectorals
Intercostal recession

3 ↑Heart rate
4 ↓ Ability to talk
5 Deviated trachea if tension pneumothorax
6 Cyanosis
7 Clammy, sweating
8 Confused

} In life- threatening attacks

9 Pulsus paradoxus

Obligate investigations in all severe asthma

- CXR (every severe attack)
- ABG (repeated as long as sick)

Stepwise approach to asthma therapy (adult)

Based on British Thoracic Society guidelines, 2009, update brit-thoracic.org.uk/

Move down to the lowest step for adequate control
Move up to improve control (but review compliance)

Inhaled short-acting β2-agonist as required

Mild and intermittent asthma
Step 1

ADD: Inhaled low-dose steroid

Regular preventer therapy
Step 2

ADD: Inhaled long-acting β2-agonist
If improvement but still poor control, increase inhaled steroid (to 800 µg/day)
If no improvement, increase steroid and trial leukotriene receptor antagonist or SR theophyline

Initial add-on therapy
Step 3

Consider trials of:
Increased inhaled steroid to high dose 2000 mg/day
Addition of 4th drug: leukotriene receptor antagonist
SR theophyline
oral β2-agonist

Persistent poor control
Step 4

ADD: Oral steroid, lowest dose possible
Maintain high-dose inhaled steroid
Consider other treatments to minimize use of oral steroids
Refer to specialist

Frequent oral steroid
Step 5

Control of asthma is defined as:
- No daytime symptoms
- No need for rescue medication
- No limitations on activity
- No night-time awakening due to asthma
- No exacerbations
- Normal lung function

Asthma remains a common chronic condition which may have life-threatening exacerbations if not treated promptly. This chapter covers the presentation and management of the disease.

Definition

There is no universally accepted definition. Asthma is present if a combination of cough, wheeze or breathlessness with *variable* airflow obstruction is present.

Epidemiology

Asthma is the single most important cause of respiratory disease morbidity and causes 2000 deaths/year in the UK. The prevalence, currently 10–15%, is increasing in western societies. The incidence of wheeze is highest in childhood (one in three children wheeze and one in seven schoolchildren have a diagnosis of asthma). Asthma is classified as:

• **Extrinsic** – childhood asthma, associated with atopy (atopy = familial allergic diathesis, manifest as childhood eczema and hay fever); it often remits by teenage years, although it may recur during adult life
• **Intrinsic** – develops in later life, is less likely to be caused by allergy, may be more progressive and does not respond as well to treatment
• **Occupational** – relates to industrial / work place allergens (e.g. photocopier material, baking, soldering, welding, paint spraying)

Aetiology

Genetics

Asthma runs in families in association with atopy. Genetic studies show a linkage to the high-affinity IgE receptor and the T-helper (Th2) cytokine genes (chromosome 5).

Environmental factors

Specific bronchial stimuli include house-dust mite, pollen and cat dander; 3% of the population is sensitive to aspirin.

• **Occupational exposure** to irritants or sensitizers is an important cause of work-related asthma
• **Non-specific stimuli**, such as viral infections, cold air, exercise or emotional stress, may also precipitate wheeze. High atmospheric levels of ozone (e.g. as found during a thunderstorm) or particulate matter predispose to exacerbations of pre-existing asthma
• **Other environmental factors**, including dietary ones (high Na^+, low $Mg2^+$), reduced incidence of childhood infections (partly as a result of immunization) and increased environmental load of allergens (dust mite), are responsible for increasing prevalence

Pathology

Airway remodelling occurs with smooth muscle hypertrophy and fibrosis. Histology shows inflammatory cell infiltrates (particularly eosinophils) in airway walls.

Clinical features

Asthma presents with symptoms of cough, wheeze and breathlessness, which vary over time (Fig. 34.1). An obvious trigger such as exercise or allergen exposure may be present. Examination may be normal or may reveal expiratory wheeze.

Assessment

Lung function Primary assessment is with spirometry. Asthma is probable when inhaled bronchodilators cause more than 15% improvement in forced expiratory volume in 1 second (FEV_1) or peak expiratory flow rate (PEFR). The absence of improvement does not rule out asthma – the patient could be in remission and chronic severe asthma is poorly reversible. Airway resistance is least at midday and greatest at 3–4 a.m. Serial measurements of PEFR in the morning, mid-day and on retiring are useful for identifying the enhanced variation in airflow limitation characteristic of asthma and for assessing response to therapy over time. Poorly controlled asthma shows a characteristic morning fall in PEFR (**morning dipping**). Occupational asthma is suggested when PEFR improves after a break from work. Lung function tests are often coupled with exercise tests in children, who often exhibit exercise-induced asthma.

Bronchial provocation tests These can determine **hyperresponsiveness** when asthma is suspected but spirometry is not diagnostic. Patients inhale increasing doses of histamine or methacholine (acetylcholine analogue) until FEV_1 declines by 20%. The dose at which this occurs (PD_{20} FEV_1) is greatly reduced in asthmatics, who are always hyperresponsive.

Skin prick tests These identify extrinsic factors. The development of a wheal around the prick site indicates allergen sensitivity. Exposure to identified allergens should be minimized (e.g. replacement of furnishings to reduce house dust mite, removal of pets). Only 50% of patients with occupational asthma are cured by the avoidance of precipitating factors.

Poorly controlled asthma This is often related to poor compliance with treatment regimens (e.g. due to peer pressure in children). Poor inhaler techniques are common. Compliance may also be poor when asthma is apparently controlled, so patients stop preventer therapies (e.g. steroids) because they are 'cured'. Patient education and training are therefore key to asthma therapy.

Severe uncontrolled asthma

This requires immediate treatment and hospitalization.
• **Indications** – inability to complete sentences ('telegraph speaking'), high respiratory rate, tachycardia and PEFR < 50% predicted
• Becomes **life-threatening** with one or more of: PEFR < 33% predicted, hypoxaemia, hypercapnia, silent chest, exhaustion
• **Treatment** – immediate nebulized β_2-agonists ± ipratropium delivered in oxygen and IV steroids, with subsequent oral steroids. In unresolving cases, IV β_2-agonists or xanthines and ventilation may be required

Prognosis

Asthma is a chronic disease requiring maintenance treatment. If asthma is not adequately treated with inhaled corticosteroids, lung function is liable to deteriorate over time and airflow obstruction may become irreversible. Risk factors for death from asthma include poor treatment compliance, ITU admissions and hospital admission despite steroid treatment.

TOP TIPS

• Family history is very important
• Look for trigger causes of exacerbations
• Explain need for long-term follow up and regular therapy
• Use stepwise progression to drug therapy in treatment
• Keep patient and carers aware of management plans

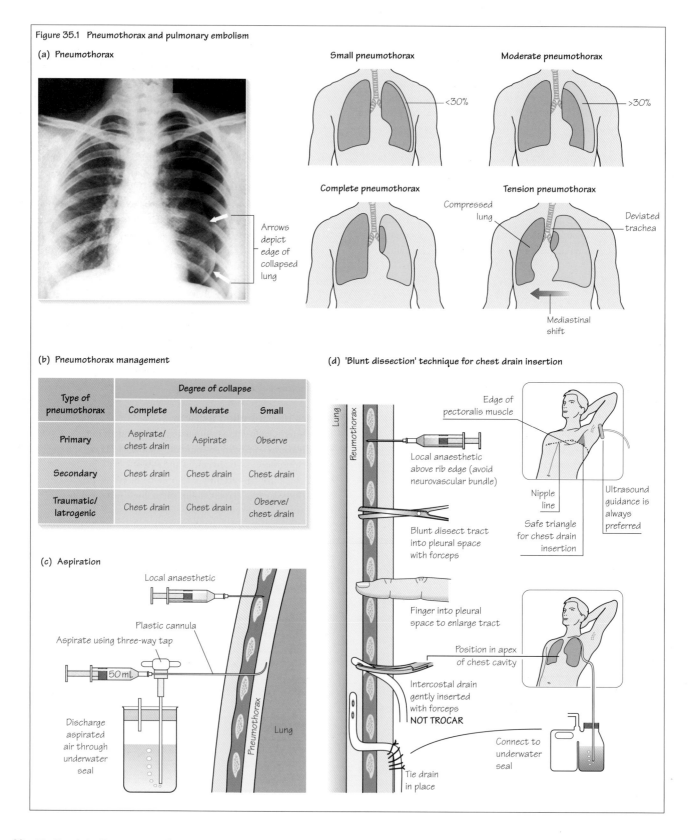

Figure 35.1 Pneumothorax and pulmonary embolism

(a) Pneumothorax

Small pneumothorax — <30%

Moderate pneumothorax — >30%

Arrows depict edge of collapsed lung

Complete pneumothorax

Tension pneumothorax

Compressed lung

Deviated trachea

Mediastinal shift

(b) Pneumothorax management

Type of pneumothorax	Degree of collapse		
	Complete	Moderate	Small
Primary	Aspirate/chest drain	Aspirate	Observe
Secondary	Chest drain	Chest drain	Chest drain
Traumatic/Iatrogenic	Chest drain	Chest drain	Observe/chest drain

(c) Aspiration

Local anaesthetic

Plastic cannula

Aspirate using three-way tap

50 mL

Discharge aspirated air through underwater seal

Pneumothorax

Lung

(d) 'Blunt dissection' technique for chest drain insertion

Lung

Pneumothorax

Local anaesthetic above rib edge (avoid neurovascular bundle)

Blunt dissect tract into pleural space with forceps

Finger into pleural space to enlarge tract

Intercostal drain gently inserted with forceps NOT TROCAR

Tie drain in place

Edge of pectoralis muscle

Nipple line

Safe triangle for chest drain insertion

Ultrasound guidance is always preferred

Position in apex of chest cavity

Connect to underwater seal

This chapter covers the presentation and management of two acute, potentially life-threatening, clinical events.

Pneumothorax

Definition

A pneumothorax is a collection of air between the visceral and parietal pleura causing a real rather than potential pleural space. Recognition and early drainage can be life saving. Predisposing and precipitating factors include necrotizing lung pathology, chest trauma, ventilator-associated lung injury and cardiothoracic surgery.

Classification

Primary spontaneous pneumothorax (PSP)

This is caused by the rupture of small apical subpleural air cysts ('blebs') but rarely causes significant physiological disturbance. Tall young (20–40 years old) men (male:female 5:1) with no underlying lung disease are usually affected. It is the most common type of pneumothorax (prevalence 8/105 per year, rising to 200/105 per year in subjects > 1.9 m in height).

Secondary pneumothorax (SP)

This is associated with respiratory diseases that damage the lung architecture, most commonly obstructive (e.g. chronic obstructive pulmonary disease (COPD), asthma), fibrotic or infective (e.g. pneumonia), and occasionally rare or inherited disorders (e.g. Marfan's, cystic fibrosis). The incidence of SP increases with age and the severity of the underlying lung disease.

Traumatic (iatrogenic) pneumothorax

This follows blunt (e.g. road traffic accidents) or penetrating (e.g. fractured ribs, stab wounds) chest trauma. Therapeutic procedures (e.g. line insertion, thoracic surgery) are common causes of iatrogenic pneumothorax.

Tension pneumothorax

A tension pneumothorax may complicate PSP or SP but is most common during mechanical ventilation and following traumatic pneumothorax. It occurs when air accumulates in the pleural cavity faster than it can be removed. Increased intrathoracic pressure causes mediastinal shift, compression of the functioning lung, inhibition of venous return and shock due to reduced cardiac output. It is a medical emergency and fatal if not rapidly relieved by drainage. Detection is a clinical diagnosis; awaiting chest X-ray (CXR) confirmation may be life threatening. Immediate drainage with a 14 G needle in the second intercostal space in the midclavicular line is essential. A characteristic 'hiss' of escaping gas confirms the diagnosis. A chest drain is then inserted.

Assessment

Pneumothorax is graded and treated as shown in Fig. 35.1. Sudden breathlessness and/or sharp pleuritic pain suggests a pneumothorax. Most PSPs are small (< 30%) and cause few symptoms other than pain. Clinical signs can be surprisingly difficult to detect, but in larger pneumothoraxes reduced air entry and hyperresonant percussion over one hemithorax are characteristic and may be associated with tachypnoea and cyanosis. Cardiorespiratory compromise may develop remarkably quickly in a tension pneumothorax and requires immediate drainage. Occasionally, other pulmonary air leaks may occur. **Monitoring** reveals tachycardia, hypotension and desaturation. **Blood gases** may demonstrate respiratory failure. **CXR** confirms the diagnosis (Fig. 35.1a). **CT scan** may detect localized pneumothoraces.

Management

Immediate supportive therapy includes supplemental oxygen and analgesia. Treatment is dependent on the cause, size and symptoms.

A tension pneumothorax must be drained immediately. A small PSP (< 30%) is simply observed and spontaneous reabsorption is confirmed on serial outpatient CXRs. A PSP > 30% may be aspirated through a 16 G needle in the second intercostal space in the midclavicular line, using a 50 mL syringe connected to a three-way tap and underwater seal (Fig. 35.1c). Following overnight observation, successful aspiration is confirmed by lung re-expansion on a repeat CXR. Occasionally, intercostal tube drainage is required for a large PSP with respiratory failure or if aspiration is unsuccessful.

In general, SP and traumatic pneumothoraxes *always* require hospital admission and intercostal chest drain insertion (Fig. 35.1d). Multiple intercostal drains may be needed to ensure adequate lung re-expansion in some patients with multiple loculated pneumothoraces. In mechanically ventilated patients, high airway pressures or large tidal volumes encourage persistent leaks and must be avoided.

Small chest drains (16 G) are nearly always adequate. Large chest drains are painful and have no significant benefits.

A persistent drain leak suggests development of a **bronchopleural fistula** (BPF). High-flow wall suction with pressures of 5–50 cmH$_2$O may oppose visceral and parietal pleura, allowing spontaneous pleurodesis. Physiotherapy and bronchial toilette are required to maintain airway patency. Early advice on surgical BPF management is essential. Video-assisted thoracoscopy is as effective as thoracotomy at correcting BPF but causes less respiratory dysfunction.

Chest drains are removed when CXR confirms lung expansion and there has been no air leakage through the drain for more than 24 hours. Drains should not be clamped before removal. Following adequate analgesia, the drain is pulled out when the patient is in inspiration. Pursestring sutures around the drainage site are then tightly secured.

Pulmonary embolism

Definition

Pulmonary embolisms (PEs) result when thrombi (often from the deep veins of the thigh or pelvis) embolize via the right heart into the pulmonary arteries.

Risk factors

Predisposing factors are found in 90% of patients and are an important clue to diagnosis. They comprise:

- Surgery less than 12 weeks ago
- Immobilization for more than 3 days in the last 4 weeks
- Previous deep venous thrombosis (DVT)/ PE or family history
- Lower limb fracture
- Malignancy
- Postpartum
- Long-distance travel, especially in cramped conditions

Pneumothorax and pulmonary embolism (continued)

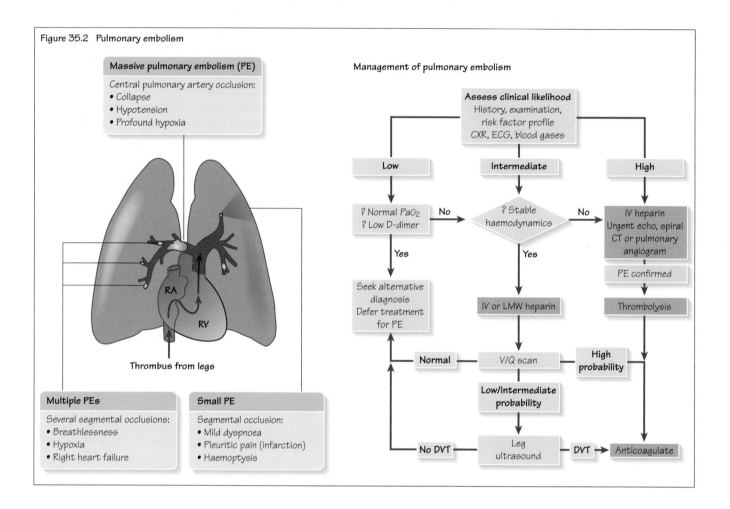

Figure 35.2   Pulmonary embolism

Massive pulmonary embolism (PE)

Central pulmonary artery occlusion:
- Collapse
- Hypotension
- Profound hypoxia

RA

RV

Thrombus from legs

Multiple PEs

Several segmental occlusions:
- Breathlessness
- Hypoxia
- Right heart failure

Small PE

Segmental occlusion:
- Mild dyspnoea
- Pleuritic pain (infarction)
- Haemoptysis

Management of pulmonary embolism

Assess clinical likelihood
History, examination,
risk factor profile
CXR, ECG, blood gases

Low | Intermediate | High

? Normal PaO$_2$
? Low D-dimer → No

? Stable haemodynamics → No

IV heparin
Urgent echo, spiral
CT or pulmonary
angiogram

PE confirmed

Yes

Yes

Seek alternative
diagnosis
Defer treatment
for PE

IV or LMW heparin

Thrombolysis

Normal

V/Q scan

High
probability

Low/intermediate
probability

No DVT

Leg
ultrasound

DVT → Anticoagulate

Clinical features

The clinical presentation of PE can be varied, so a high degree of clinical suspicion is required. PEs cause hypoxia from ventilation/perfusion ($\dot{V}/\dot{Q}$) mismatch and interrupt pulmonary blood flow, causing pulmonary infarcts (so inflaming the pleura) and lowering cardiac output (Fig. 35.2). These features are responsible for the three distinct clinical syndromes with which pulmonary thromboembolic disease presents:

1 Pleurisy and/or haemoptysis – small or moderate-sized PEs cause pulmonary infarction. Dyspnoea is absent or minor.

2 Dyspnoea with hypoxia in the absence of other causes – this suggests a moderate or large PE or repeated PEs over a period of time. There may be signs of cardiopulmonary disturbance (tachycardia, tachypnoea, elevated jugular venous pressure (JVP), left parasternal lift from acute right heart strain). Pleurisy/haemoptysis is often absent.

3 Circulatory collapse – large or massive PE. Typically a high-risk patient (e.g. post-surgery) with unheralded collapse or unexplained clinical deterioration, and with hypotension, tachycardia and hypoxia.

Investigations

An assessment of the likelihood of PE, based on clinical, blood gas and CXR parameters remains central to the diagnosis of PE, and directs early therapy. Later therapy is guided by more specific tests, e.g. $\dot{V}/\dot{Q}$ scans, although these often suggest rather than confirm the diagnosis.

Treatment (Fig. 35.2)

- **Oxygen**: should be given to all patients with suspected PE
- **Heparin**: should be administered when there is clinical suspicion of PE, while investigations are completed. IV heparin should be used for large or massive PE, and subcutaneous low molecular weight (LMW) heparin in small or moderate PE
- **Thrombolysis**: streptokinase or tissue plasminogen activator (tPA) dissolves thrombi. It is indicated for confirmed PE with hypotension, severe hypoxia or other evidence of marked haemodynamic compromise
- **Warfarin**: initial treatment with heparin should be followed by oral anticoagulation with warfarin once the diagnosis of PE is confirmed, aiming for an international normalized ratio (INR) of 2.5–3.0. If there is a remediable underlying cause (e.g. surgery, immobility), anticoagulation for 6 weeks is adequate. If not, the incidence of recurrent PE is high, so anticoagulation should be continued for longer, often indefinitely.

TOP TIPS

- Sudden onset breathlessness and pain – think pneumothorax
- Take a full history of recent operations or traumatology
- Confirm diagnosis quickly but do not wait to give symptomatic relief
- Think risk factors for PE

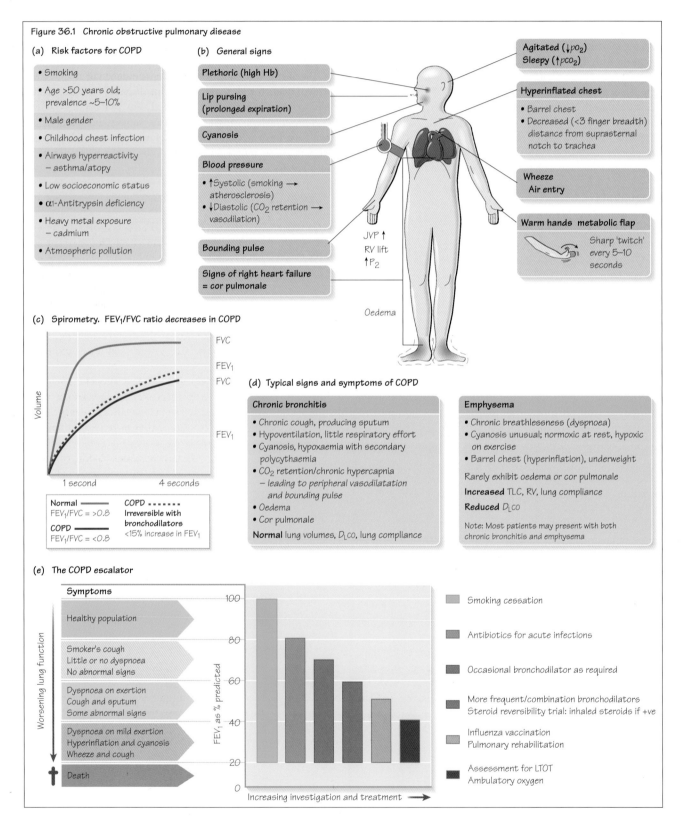

Figure 36.1 Chronic obstructive pulmonary disease

(a) Risk factors for COPD

- Smoking
- Age >50 years old; prevalence ~5–10%
- Male gender
- Childhood chest infection
- Airways hyperreactivity – asthma/atopy
- Low socioeconomic status
- α1-Antitrypsin deficiency
- Heavy metal exposure – cadmium
- Atmospheric pollution

(b) General signs

- Plethoric (high Hb)
- Lip pursing (prolonged expiration)
- Cyanosis

Blood pressure
- ↑Systolic (smoking → atherosclerosis)
- ↓Diastolic (CO_2 retention → vasodilation)

Bounding pulse

Signs of right heart failure = cor pulmonale

Agitated (↓po_2)
Sleepy (↑pco_2)

Hyperinflated chest
- Barrel chest
- Decreased (<3 finger breadth) distance from suprasternal notch to trachea

Wheeze
Air entry

Warm hands metabolic flap
Sharp 'twitch' every 5–10 seconds

JVP ↑
RV lift
↑P_2

Oedema

(c) Spirometry. FEV_1/FVC ratio decreases in COPD

FVC
FEV_1
FVC
FEV_1

Volume

1 second   4 seconds

Normal —— FEV_1/FVC = >0.8
COPD —— FEV_1/FVC = <0.8

COPD ·······
Irreversible with bronchodilators
<15% increase in FEV_1

(d) Typical signs and symptoms of COPD

Chronic bronchitis
- Chronic cough, producing sputum
- Hypoventilation, little respiratory effort
- Cyanosis, hypoxaemia with secondary polycythaemia
- CO_2 retention/chronic hypercapnia – leading to peripheral vasodilatation and bounding pulse
- Oedema
- Cor pulmonale

Normal lung volumes, D_LCO, lung compliance

Emphysema
- Chronic breathlessness (dyspnoea)
- Cyanosis unusual; normoxic at rest, hypoxic on exercise
- Barrel chest (hyperinflation), underweight

Rarely exhibit oedema or cor pulmonale

Increased TLC, RV, lung compliance

Reduced D_LCO

Note: Most patients may present with both chronic bronchitis and emphysema

(e) The COPD escalator

Symptoms

Worsening lung function

- Healthy population
- Smoker's cough
  Little or no dyspnoea
  No abnormal signs
- Dyspnoea on exertion
  Cough and sputum
  Some abnormal signs
- Dyspnoea on mild exertion
  Hyperinflation and cyanosis
  Wheeze and cough
- Death

FEV_1 as % predicted

Increasing investigation and treatment →

- Smoking cessation
- Antibiotics for acute infections
- Occasional bronchodilator as required
- More frequent/combination bronchodilators
  Steroid reversibility trial: inhaled steroids if +ve
- Influenza vaccination
  Pulmonary rehabilitation
- Assessment for LTOT
  Ambulatory oxygen

COPD is a major public health problem from which 30 000 people die per year in the UK (5.1% of all deaths). The prevalence is $\geq$900 000. Rates are higher in industrialized countries, in inner city areas, among lower income groups and in elderly people. Rates have reached a plateau in men but are still rising in women. This chapter covers the presentation and management of this irreversible condition (Fig. 36.1).

Definition

Chronic obstructive pulmonary disease (COPD) and chronic obstructive airway disease are interchangeable terms. It is a chronic, slowly progressive disorder characterized by fixed or partially reversible airway obstruction, unlike the reversible airway obstruction seen in asthma.

Aetiology

- **Environmental factors** – cigarette smoking is the major cause, with additional risk from atmospheric pollutants in the workplace or inner city. Some patients have chronic, undiagnosed and untreated asthma
- **Genetics** – α_1-antitrypsin deficiency predisposes to early development of COPD

Pathology

Smoking causes bronchial mucus gland hypertrophy and increased mucus production, leading to a productive cough. In chronic bronchitis ('productive cough' > 3 months/year for > 2 years) the early changes are in the small airways. In addition, destruction of lung tissue with dilatation of the distal airspaces (emphysema) occurs, leading to loss of elastic recoil, hyperinflation, gas trapping and an increase in the work of breathing, causing breathlessness. As the disease progresses CO_2 levels rise and the drive to respiration switches from CO_2 to hypoxaemia. If supplementary oxygen corrects hypoxaemia, the drive to respiration may also be removed, provoking respiratory failure.

Clinical features

Slowly progressing symptoms of cough and shortness of breath over several years in a smoker or ex-smoker suggests the diagnosis. Severity is defined according to the degree of airflow obstruction (FEV_1):
- *Mild disease*: FEV_1 50–80% of age/sex predicted – cough, minimal dyspnoea and normal examination
- *Moderate disease*: FEV_1 30–49% – cough, breathless on moderate exertion, wheeze, hyperinflation and reduced air entry
- *Severe disease*: FEV_1 < 30% – cough, breathless on minimal exertion, signs of moderate COPD and possibly of respiratory failure and cor pulmonale

Investigations

- **Pulmonary function tests** show airflow obstruction and reduced gas transfer as a result of destruction of lung tissue. Total lung capacity may be normal, or increased as a result of gas trapping. Twenty per cent of patients derive benefit from bronchodilators. Response to bronchodilator treatment is not predicted by reversibility testing, which is therefore not recommended

- **Chest X-ray** may be normal but, in emphysema, will reveal hyperinflation with loss of lung markings and a small heart
- **Computed tomography** may confirm emphysematous bullae
- **Blood gases** should be analyzed if there is any suspicion of respiratory failure. In chronic hypoxaemia the haemoglobin may be increased

Management

- **Smoking cessation** is a priority.
- **Bronchodilators** (β-agonists or anticholinergics) are used in the 20–40% who benefit. In severe disease up to 10% of patients derive more benefit if high doses are delivered by nebulizer rather than metered dose inhaler. A 2-week trial of oral steroids should be considered to determine reversibility (from serial peak flow or spirometry) of airway obstruction if a diagnosis of untreated asthma is suspected. Long-acting bronchodilators are recommended in patients who are still symptomatic on short-acting drugs and in patients with more than two exacerbations per year
- Long-term **oxygen therapy** (LTOT) for > 16 hours daily prolongs life in patients with chronic respiratory failure (i.e. those with a PaO_2 of < 7.3 kPa and FEV_1 of < 1.5 L)
- In an acute exacerbation, treatment may need to be increased. **Antibiotics** have not been shown to improve outcome, although short-course antibiotics shorten symptom duration of purulent sputum and respiratory deterioration. **Oral steroids** improve recovery from acute exacerbations. Long-term **inhaled steroids** reduce the frequency of exacerbations in those with moderate disease and should be used in those with an FEV_1 of < 50% and at least one exacerbation per year
- **Pulmonary rehabilitation** (especially exercise training) produces significant symptomatic benefit in patients with moderate to severe disease
- **Resection of large bullae** enables adjacent areas of the lung to reinflate. **Lung volume reduction surgery** may also produce improvement by improving elastic recoil, so maintaining airway patency. Selection of patients is important – currently there are no clear criteria. **Lung transplantation** is very rarely used
- **Prevention of acute COPD exacerbations** includes pneumococcal and influenza vaccination. Patients with any combination of increased dyspnoea, increased sputum or purulent sputum benefit from antibiotics targeted against common respiratory pathogens (e.g. *Haemophilus influenzae*). Short courses of oral corticosteroids improve lung function and hasten recovery in patients with acute exacerbations
- **Overall prognosis** for COPD patients is dependent on the severity of airflow obstruction. Patients with a FEV_1 < 0.8 L have a yearly mortality of approximately 25%. Patients with cor pulmonale, hypercapnia, ongoing cigarette smoking and weight loss have a worse prognosis. Death usually occurs from infection, acute respiratory failure, pulmonary embolus or cardiac arrhythmia

> **TOP TIPS**
> - Take a full history of the risk factors
> - Look for the cause of acute exacerbations
> - Involve primary care services at discharge
> - Involve carers in understanding the chronic and acute nature of the condition

Figure 37.1 Community-acquired pneumonia

(a) Pneumonia affecting the right lower lobe

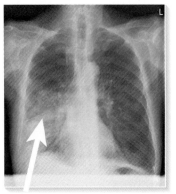

Consolidation right lower lobe

(b) Pneumonia affecting lingula lobe

Consolidation lingula lobe

(c) Risk factors for pneumonia

- Age: >65, <5 years old
- Chronic disease (e.g. renal and lung)
- Diabetes mellitus
- Immunosuppression (e.g. drugs and HIV)
- Alcohol dependency
- Aspiration (e.g. epilepsy)
- Recent viral illness (e.g. influenza)
- Malnutrition
- Mechanical ventilation
- Postoperative (e.g. obesity and smoking)
- Environmental (e.g. psittacosis)
- Occupational (e.g. Q fever)
- Travel abroad (e.g. paragonimiasis)
- Air conditioning (e.g. Legionella)

(d) Microorganisms and pathological insults that cause pneumonia

Bacterial infections	Atypical infections	Fungal infection
Streptococcus pneumoniae	Mycoplasma pneumoniae	Aspergillus
Haemophilus influenzae	Legionella pneumophila	Histoplasmosis
Klebsiella pneumoniae	Coxiella burnetii	Candida
Pseudomonas aeruginosa	Chlamydia psittaci	Nocardia
Gram-negative (E. coli)		

Viral infections	Protozoal infections	Other causes
Influenza	Pneumocystis jirovecii	Aspiration
Coxsackie	Toxoplasmosis	Lipoid pneumonia
Adenovirus	Amoebiasis	Bronchiectasis
Respiratory syncytial	Paragonimiasis	Cystic fibrosis
Cytomegalovirus		Radiation

(e) Non-hospital (i.e. community) management of CAP using the recently validated CRB-65 score

Score 1 point for each of:
- Confusion (mental test score <8 or new disorientation)
- Respiratory rate ≥30/min
- Blood pressure (SBP<90 mmHg or DBP ≤60 mmHg)
- Age ≥65 years

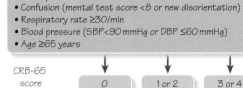

CRB-65 score (Associated mortality)

| 0 (1.2%) | 1 or 2 (5–12%) | 3 or 4 (33–48%) |

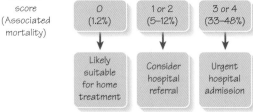

| Likely suitable for home treatment | Consider hospital referral | Urgent hospital admission |

(f) Complications and infection specific features of pneumonia

* = Rare
** = Very rare

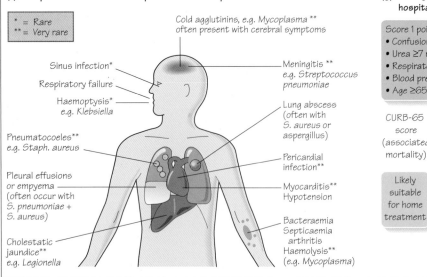

Cold agglutinins, e.g. Mycoplasma ** often present with cerebral symptoms

Sinus infection*

Respiratory failure

Haemoptysis*
e.g. Klebsiella

Pneumatocoeles**
e.g. Staph. aureus

Pleural effusions
or empyema
(often occur with
S. pneumoniae +
S. aureus)

Cholestatic
jaundice**
e.g. Legionella

Meningitis **
e.g. Streptococcus
pneumoniae

Lung abscess
(often with
S. aureus or
aspergillus)

Pericardial
infection**

Myocarditis**
Hypotension

Bacteraemia
Septicaemia
arthritis
Haemolysis**
(e.g. Mycoplasma)

(g) Management of CAP in patients admitted to hospital using the recently validated CURB-65 score

Score 1 point for each of:
- Confusion (mental test score <8 or new disorientation)
- Urea ≥7 mmol/L (i.e. includes use of laboratory tests)
- Respiratory rate >30/min
- Blood pressure (SBP<90 mmHg or DBP ≤60 mmHg)
- Age ≥65 years

CURB-65 score (associated mortality)

| 0 or 1 (1–3%) | 2 (13%) | 3 or more (17–57%) |

| Likely suitable for home treatment | Consider hospital-supervised treatment Options include: a) Short stay in-patient b) Hospital-supervised outpatient | Manage in hospital as severe pneumonia Assess for ICU admission especially if CURB-65 is >4 |

Patients admitted to hospital with pneumonia are already potentially very ill. This chapter covers the common causes and immediate assessment and management of the patient.

Pneumonia is an **acute lower respiratory tract (LRT) illness**, usually due to **infection**, associated with **fever, focal chest symptoms (±signs)** and **new shadowing on CXR** (Fig. 37.1a). Figure 37.1c lists microorganisms and pathological insults that cause pneumonia.

Classification

In the clinical situation, **microbiological classification** of pneumonia is not practical as causative organisms may not be identified and diagnosis takes several days. Likewise, **anatomical** (radiographical) appearance (e.g. lobar pneumonia (affecting one lobe) or bronchopneumonia (widespread, patchy involvement)) gives little practical information about cause. The following classification is widely accepted:

• **Community-acquired pneumonia** (CAP): describes LRT infections occurring within 48 hours of hospital admission in patients who have not been hospitalized for more than 14 days. The most frequently identified organism is *Streptococcus pneumoniae* (20–75%). *Mycoplasma pneumoniae, Chlamydia pneumoniae* and *Legionalla* spp., the 'atypical' bacterial pathogens (2–25%) and viral infections (8–12%) are relatively common causes. *Haemophilus influenzae* and *Moraxella catarrhalis* are associated with COPD exacerbations, and staphylococcal infection may follow influenza. Alcoholic, diabetic and nursing home patients are prone to infection with staphylococcal, anaerobic and Gram-negative organisms

• **Hospital-acquired (nosocomial) pneumonia**: any LRT infections developing more than 2 days after hospital admission. Likely organisms are Gram-negative bacilli (~70%) or *Staphylococcus* (~15%)

• **Aspiration/anaerobic pneumonia**: bacteroides and other anaerobic infections follow aspiration of oropharyngeal contents (e.g. CVA)

• **Opportunistic pneumonia**: immunosuppressed patients (e.g. steroids, chemotherapy, HIV) are susceptible to viral, fungal and mycobacterial infections, in addition to other bacterial organisms

Epidemiology

Annual incidence is 5–11 cases per 1000 adult population; 15–45% require hospitalization (1–4 cases per 1000) of whom 5–10% are treated in ITU. Incidence is highest in the very young and elderly. **Mortality** is 5–12% in hospitalized patients and 25–50% in ITU patients. **Seasonal variation** is seen with peaks (e.g. *Mycoplasma* in autumn, *Staphylococcus* in spring) and annual cycles (e.g. 4-yearly *Mycoplasma* epidemics). **Frequent viral infections increase CAP in winter**.

Risk factors

Factors associated with increased risk of CAP are listed in Fig. 37.1c. **Specific risk factors** include **age** (e.g. *Mycoplasma* in young adults), **occupation** (e.g. brucellosis in abattoir workers, Q fever in sheep workers), **environment** (e.g. psittacosis with pet birds, erlichiosis due to tick bites) or **geographical** (e.g. coccidiomycosis in southwest USA). Epidemics of *Coxiella burnetti* (Q fever) or *Legionella pneumophila* are often localized (e.g. Legionnaires' disease may involve a specific hotel due to air conditioner contamination).

Clinical features

These are inaccurate without a CXR and cannot predict causative organisms (i.e. 'atypical' pathogens do not have characteristic presentations). **Symptoms** may be general (e.g. malaise, fever, rigors, myalgia) or chest-specific (e.g. dyspnoea, pleurisy, cough, haemoptysis). Signs include cyanosis, tachycardia and tachypnoea; with focal dullness, crepitations, bronchial breathing and pleuritic rub on chest examination. In young or old patients and atypical pneumonias (e.g. *Mycoplasma*), non-respiratory features (e.g. confusion, rashes, diarrhoea) may predominate. Complications are shown in Fig. 36.1f.

Investigations

• FBC
• C-reactive protein
• LFTs
• Blood gases
• Blood cultures
• Chest X-rays/CT scans

Severity assessment

The following features are associated with increased mortality and indicate the need for monitoring in ITU:

• *Clinical*: age more than 60 years; respiratory rate more than 30/min; diastolic blood pressure less than 60 mmHg; new atrial fibrillation; confusion; multilobar involvement; and coexisting illness
• *Laboratory*: urea > 7 mmol/L; albumin < 35 g/L; hypoxaemia PO_2 < 8 kPa; leucopenia (white cell count (WCC) < 4×10^9/L); leucocytosis (WCC > 20×10^9/L); and bacteraemia

Severity scoring uses CRB-65 and CURB-65 scores, which allocate points for confusion, urea > 7 mmol/L, respiratory rate > 30/min, low systolic (< 90 mmHg) or diastolic (< 60 mmHg) blood pressure and age more than 65 years. This stratifies patients into mortality groups suitable for different management pathways (Fig. 36.1e, g).

Management

Supportive measures include oxygen to maintain a PaO_2 of more than 8 kPa (SaO_2 < 90%) and intravenous fluid (± inotrope) resuscitation to ensure haemodynamic stability. Non-invasive (e.g. continuous positive airway pressure (CPAP)) or mechanical ventilation may be required in respiratory failure. Physiotherapy and bronchoscopy aid sputum clearance.

Initial antibiotic therapy should be based on the 'best guess', according to pneumonia classification and likely organisms, as microbiological results are not available for 12–72 hours. Therapy is adjusted when results and antibiotic sensitivities become available. The American and British Thoracic Societies (ATS, BTS) recommend the following initial antibiotic protocols for CAP:

• *Non-hospitalized patients*: usually respond to oral therapy with amoxicillin (BTS) or an advanced macrolide (e.g. clarithromycin) or doxycycline (ATS). Patients with severe symptoms or at risk for drug-resistant *Streptococcus pneumoniae* (e.g. recent antibiotics and co-morbidity) are treated with a β-lactam plus a macrolide or doxycycline, or an antipneumococcal fluoroquinolone (e.g. moxifloxacin) alone
• *Hospitalized patients*: initial therapy must cover 'atypical' organisms and *S. pneumoniae*. An intravenous macrolide is combined with a β-lactam or an antipneumococcal fluoroquinolone (ATS/BTS) or cefuroxime (BTS). If not severe, combined ampicillin and macrolide (oral or IV) may be adequate (BTS). Staphylococcal infection following influenza and *H. influenzae* in COPD should be covered

TOP TIPS

• Use CRB-65 and CURB-65 on admission
• Think of co-morbidities
• Remember occupational factors in younger patients
• Take drug history and allergies
• Review regularly for ongoing complications due to disease or treatment
• Keep patient and carers informed of management

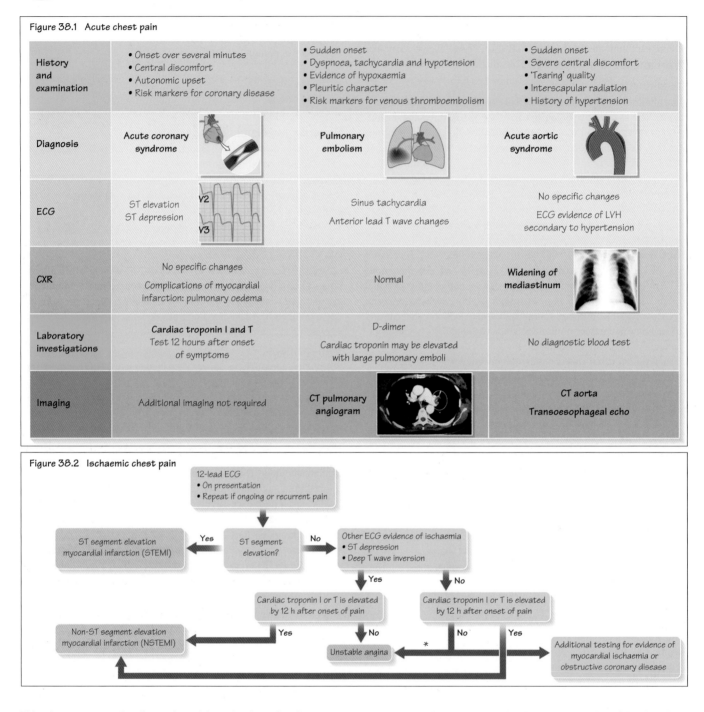

Figure 38.1 Acute chest pain

History and examination	• Onset over several minutes • Central discomfort • Autonomic upset • Risk markers for coronary disease	• Sudden onset • Dyspnoea, tachycardia and hypotension • Evidence of hypoxaemia • Pleuritic character • Risk markers for venous thromboembolism	• Sudden onset • Severe central discomfort • 'Tearing' quality • Interscapular radiation • History of hypertension
Diagnosis	Acute coronary syndrome	Pulmonary embolism	Acute aortic syndrome
ECG	ST elevation ST depression	Sinus tachycardia Anterior lead T wave changes	No specific changes ECG evidence of LVH secondary to hypertension
CXR	No specific changes Complications of myocardial infarction: pulmonary oedema	Normal	Widening of mediastinum
Laboratory investigations	Cardiac troponin I and T Test 12 hours after onset of symptoms	D-dimer Cardiac troponin may be elevated with large pulmonary emboli	No diagnostic blood test
Imaging	Additional imaging not required	CT pulmonary angiogram	CT aorta Transoesophageal echo

Figure 38.2 Ischaemic chest pain

12-lead ECG
• On presentation
• Repeat if ongoing or recurrent pain

ST segment elevation? — Yes → ST segment elevation myocardial infarction (STEMI)

ST segment elevation? — No → Other ECG evidence of ischaemia
• ST depression
• Deep T wave inversion

Other ECG evidence of ischaemia — Yes → Cardiac troponin I or T is elevated by 12 h after onset of pain

Other ECG evidence of ischaemia — No → Cardiac troponin I or T is elevated by 12 h after onset of pain

Cardiac troponin I or T is elevated by 12 h after onset of pain (left) — Yes → Non-ST segment elevation myocardial infarction (NSTEMI)

Cardiac troponin I or T is elevated by 12 h after onset of pain (left) — No → Unstable angina

Cardiac troponin I or T is elevated by 12 h after onset of pain (right) — No → * Unstable angina

Cardiac troponin I or T is elevated by 12 h after onset of pain (right) — Yes → Additional testing for evidence of myocardial ischaemia or obstructive coronary disease

This chapter covers the diagnosis and investigation of patients presenting with acute chest pain. Acute chest pain accounts for 6% of attendances and up to 40% of emergency admissions in the UK. The goals are to detect disease such as acute myocardial infarction and discharge patients without life-threatening pathology safely.

Key points

• Acute chest pain is a medical emergency. The objective is to rapidly identify or exclude serious pathology

• A targeted history and examination combined with 12-lead ECG can be completed in 10 minutes and will lead to a diagnosis or identification of the requirement for further investigation (Fig. 38.1)

• Acute coronary syndrome patients who have ongoing pain accompanied by ST elevation on their ECG require immediate reperfusion therapy. Primary angioplasty is the treatment of choice but if the delay to angioplasty balloon inflation is greater than 90–120 minutes, thrombolysis should be considered

• The early mortality from dissection affecting the ascending aorta is high and prompt recognition with corrective surgery is key

- Patients with a pulmonary cause for chest discomfort will usually have prominent dyspnoea although this symptom will frequently be present in patients presenting with myocardial ischaemia

Differential diagnosis

Any organ within the chest may give rise to chest pain.

Heart and aorta
- Acute coronary syndromes: this umbrella term refers to patients presenting with ischaemic chest pain
- Acute aortic syndromes: an umbrella term including aortic dissection, aortic intramural haematoma and thoracic aortic aneurysm
- Pericarditis and myocarditis

Lung
- Pulmonary embolism (PE)
- Pneumonia
- Pneumothorax

Oesophagus, stomach and abdominal disease
- Gastroesophageal reflux disease (GORD)
- Peptic ulcer disease
- Oesophageal dysmotility disorders
- Abdominal pathology, e.g. splenic infarction

Chest wall
- Costochondritis
- Inflammatory or degenerative joint disease affecting the chest wall or thoracic spine, e.g. ankylosing spondylitis, osteoarthritis
- Herpes zoster

Important diagnostic features

Ischaemic chest pain
- Central location with radiation across the chest. Radiation to the arms, neck and jaw is common. Ischaemic pain may be isolated in the epigastric region, shoulder, arm or neck
- Patients often describe a 'discomfort', 'ache', 'tightness' or 'heaviness' in preference to using the word 'pain'. The discomfort may be mild. Some patients with myocardial infarction may be asymptomatic or have symptoms of nausea or dyspnoea alone. These atypical presentations are more common in the elderly and patients with diabetes
- A past medical history of angina, established vascular disease such as stroke and risk markers for coronary disease such as diabetes heighten suspicion of an acute coronary syndrome
- Patients with antecedent angina will often describe a clear relationship with exertion and relief with rest and glyceryl trinitrate spray

Pulmonary embolism
- The absence of dyspnoea makes this diagnosis unlikely
- Often evidence of hypoxia but normal O_2 sats possible

Pleuritic pain
- Often sharp. Brought on or exacerbated by deep inspiration

Aortic dissection
- Involving the ascending aorta and arch and will often be accompanied by signs of major vessel compromise such as ischaemic stroke leading to hemiparesis or limb ischaemia
- Involvement of the aortic root leads to aortic regurgitation

Pericarditis
- The pain of pericarditis has pleuritic features and may be worse on inspiration and relieved by sitting forward
- ECG may demonstrate diffuse ST elevation across all ECG leads
- An elevated troponin indicates associated myocarditis

Oesophageal pain
- The typical symptom of heartburn related to GORD is easily recognized but oesophageal disease may also mimic ischaemic chest pain

Musculoskeletal pain
- Symptoms occur on chest wall movement or pressure

The acute coronary syndromes

Patients presenting with ischaemic chest discomfort at rest without diagnostic ECG changes or elevation in cardiac troponin remain at risk of death and myocardial infarction. Where there is diagnostic doubt, additional testing is performed to identify the presence of obstructive coronary disease or inducible myocardial ischaemia (Fig. 38.2).

Key investigations

ECG
- The pivotal test for identifying patients with ST elevation who need immediate reperfusion therapy
- Non-ST segment elevation myocardial infarction (NSTEMI) patients with evidence of ischaemia on the ECG are at high risk of further infarction and death and will usually require invasive coronary angiography

Cardiac troponin
- A specific marker for cardiomyocyte injury capable of detecting microscopic areas of infarction
- Further risk of infarction and death with elevated troponin
- May be a marker of intracoronary thrombus with ischaemic chest pain

Troponin elevation may be observed in other conditions associated with chest pain and cardiomyocyte injury, e.g. PE, perimyocarditis and aortic dissection

Other blood tests
- Arterial blood gas analysis
- D-dimer: a normal result makes pulmonary embolism very unlikely

Chest X-ray
- Acute aortic syndromes (widening of the mediastinum)
- Pulmonary causes of chest pain (pneumonia and pneumothorax)

CT scanning
- Useful to detect PE and acute aortic syndrome
- Coronary calcification can be detected and is a marker of atherosclerotic plaque burden in patients with coronary disease. Absence of coronary calcification makes an acute coronary syndrome unlikely

Echocardiography
- Transthoracic echo can be performed rapidly at the bedside. It often helps diagnosis but is not specific enough to exclude pathology
- Acute aortic regurgitation and a dissection flap can be seen in patients with aortic dissection. Transoesophageal echo is more sensitive and may be used as an alternative to CT scanning in these patients
- Right heart dilatation and strain may be seen in patients with PE

> **TOP TIPS**
>
> - The patient history and description of chest pain are key
> - The 12-lead ECG should be reviewed within 10 minutes of presentation and repeated in patients with further episodes of pain
> - Cardiac troponin allows risk stratification in patients presenting with ischaemic chest pain but should not be used as a screening test in patients without chest pain
> - CT scanning may be required to exclude life-threatening aortic pathology and pulmonary embolism

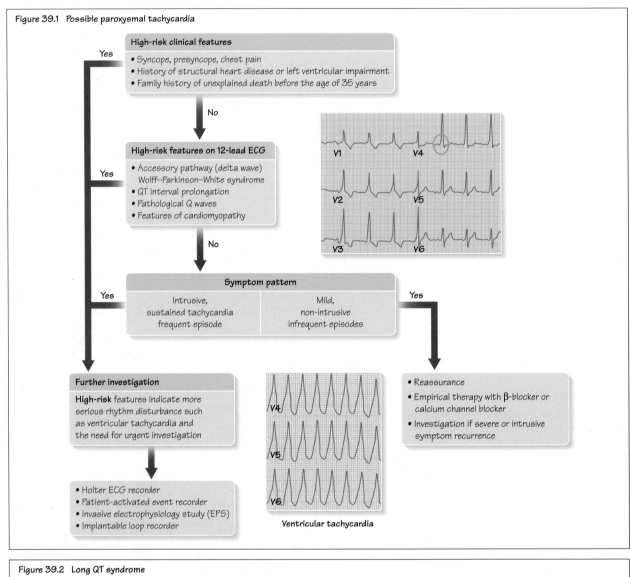

Figure 39.1 Possible paroxysmal tachycardia

High-risk clinical features

- Syncope, presyncope, chest pain
- History of structural heart disease or left ventricular impairment
- Family history of unexplained death before the age of 35 years

High-risk features on 12-lead ECG

- Accessory pathway (delta wave) Wolff–Parkinson–White syndrome
- QT interval prolongation
- Pathological Q waves
- Features of cardiomyopathy

V1 V4
V2 V5
V3 V6

Symptom pattern

| Intrusive, sustained tachycardia frequent episode | Mild, non-intrusive infrequent episodes |

Further investigation

High-risk features indicate more serious rhythm disturbance such as ventricular tachycardia and the need for urgent investigation

- Holter ECG recorder
- Patient-activated event recorder
- Invasive electrophysiology study (EPS)
- Implantable loop recorder

V4
V5
V6

Ventricular tachycardia

- Reassurance
- Empirical therapy with β-blocker or calcium channel blocker
- Investigation if severe or intrusive symptom recurrence

Figure 39.2 Long QT syndrome

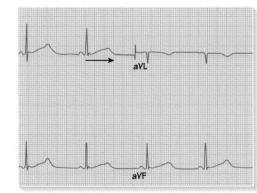

aVL

aVF

- The ECG of patients presenting with palpitation should be examined for evidence of a prolonged QT interval. This is a marker of susceptibility to ventricular tachyarrhythmias and sudden cardiac death.
- The interval (QT) is dependent on heart rate and the measured interval may be corrected (QTc) for heart rate (R to R interval) using the formula:

$$QT_c = \frac{QT}{\sqrt{RR}}$$

- A QTc greater than 450 msec is abnormal but this may be present in 2.5% of the healthy population. Equally 15% of patients with long QT syndrome may exhibit a normal QT interval.
- Long QT syndrome can arise from mutation of several genes that govern ventricular depolarisation
- QT prolongation is associated with electrolyte disturbance (↓K, ↓Mg, ↓Ca) and hypothyroidism. Many drugs prolong the QT interval including sotalol, clarithromycin, methadone, amiodarone and several antipsychotics.

This chapter covers the diagnosis and investigation of patients presenting with abnormal sensation of the heart beat or palpitations. Patients and doctors may differ in their understanding of this term. Whereas the medical use is restricted to an intrusive awareness of the heart beat, patients may use the term when describing dyspnoea or a feeling of fright and panic. Palpitation is therefore too vague a term to be clinically useful and care should be taken to understand the nature of the symptom the patient is describing. Palpitation has a high prevalence and is a common cause for presentation in primary care and referral to cardiology outpatient clinics.

Key points
- Patients with palpitation have a spectrum of underlying problems ranging from trivial to life threatening in severity
- If paroxysmal tachycardia or rhythm disturbance are suspected a 12-lead ECG should be performed at first contact
- Documenting the heart rhythm during a symptom episode is key and can prove challenging in patients with infrequent symptoms
- The initial approach involves risk stratifying patients for the possibility of life-threatening cardiac rhythm disorders. Patients with high-risk features merit urgent investigation
- The likelihood of serious underlying arrhythmia and intrusiveness of the symptom dictate the extent of investigation and treatment

Differential diagnosis: what is the patient describing?

Irregular heart beat
Patients describe 'skipped' or 'missed' beats, 'The heart stops and starts,' 'I feel a thump in my chest', 'My heart beat is all over the place.' These experiences can be due to:
- Ectopic beats
- Non-sustained tachycardia
- (Paroxysmal) atrial fibrillation

Paroxysmal tachycardia (Fig 39.1)
the sudden onset of a sustained (> 30 seconds) rapid heart beat is due to:
- Supraventricular tachycardia:
  - atrioventricular node-dependent re-entrant tachycardia (AVNRT)
  - atrioventricular re-entrant tachycardia (AVRT)
  - atrial tachycardia
  - Wolff –Parkinson–White syndrome
- Atrial flutter
- Ventricular tachycardia

Abnormal or increased awareness of the normal heartbeat
This typically has a gradual onset and occurs at quiet times, e.g. just before falling asleep. The patient's heart rate is normal or slightly increased. Common causes are:
- Anxiety and stress
- Hyperdynamic circulation, e.g. pregnancy, anaemia, hyperthyroidism, aortic regurgitation

Important diagnostic features

Supraventricular tachycardias
Patients sometimes describe polyuria in association with the tachycardia reflecting increased atrial natriuretic peptide release during the episode. Patients with AVNRT and AVRT may describe bending over as a precipitating factor. These tachycardias involve the atrioventricular node and the patient may have learned techniques to terminate the tachycardia, such as exhaling forcibly against closed lips and a pinched nose. This Valsalva manoeuvre can be taught to the patient to terminate the tachycardia.

Ventricular tachycardia
The possibility of this life-threatening rhythm disturbance should be considered if the patient describes syncope or has a past history of myocardial infarction, heart failure or structural heart disease. A family history of sudden cardiac death indicates an inherited propensity to ventricular arrhythmia such as the long QT syndrome (Fig. 39.2).

Paroxysmal atrial fibrillation
This is more common in elderly patients with hypertension and established heart disease. Patients often have sustained symptom episodes lasting longer than 30 minutes. Patients frequently report dyspnoea and reduced exercise capacity in association with palpitation, but syncope is uncommon.

Key investigations

ECG
- Patients with a history of palpitation will frequently have a normal ECG. They should be encouraged to present again for an ECG during a symptom episode if they encounter further sustained palpitation
- The 12-lead ECG should be examined for evidence of an accessory conduction pathway through the atrioventricular ring indicative of Wolf–Parkinson–White syndrome. This manifests on the ECG as a slurred upstroke in the QRS complex
- QT interval prolongation (Fig. 39.2).
- Q waves indicate previous myocardial infarction. Patients with underlying cardiomyopathy will have abnormalities such as left ventricular hypertrophy. These findings should prompt further imaging (echocardiography) to evaluate the presence of structural heart problems associated with ventricular tachycardia including left ventricular dysfunction and arrhythmogenic right ventricular dysplasia

Holter (ambulatory) ECG recorders
- The aim is to document cardiac rhythm during a symptom episode
- It is essential to correlate rhythm disturbance with symptoms as asymptomatic abnormalities including ventricular ectopics and short bursts of atrial fibrillation or atrial ectopic beats (less than 5 seconds) are common
- Documentation of normal rhythm during a symptom episode is helpful, suggesting either abnormal awareness of the heart beat or an alternative cause of the symptom
- Patient-activated recorders may be worn for 1 month, but capturing a symptom episode by holter recording often proves elusive

Invasive electrophysiology study
This is used:
- To identify causes of paroxysmal tachycardia when non-invasive studies have been unsuccessful
- For the definitive treatment of Wolf–Parkinson–White syndrome, AVNRT, AVRT, atrial flutter and atrial fibrillation by radiofrequency ablation

---

TOP TIPS

- Documenting an underlying paroxysmal rhythm disturbance with holter rhythm recorders can prove challenging
- Patients with recurrent prolonged symptom episodes should be encouraged to attend hospital when symptomatic in order to have a 12-lead ECG
- Risk stratification can readily be done to identify patients at risk of serious or life-threatening arrhythmia from the history, 12-lead ECG and cardiac imaging if necessary

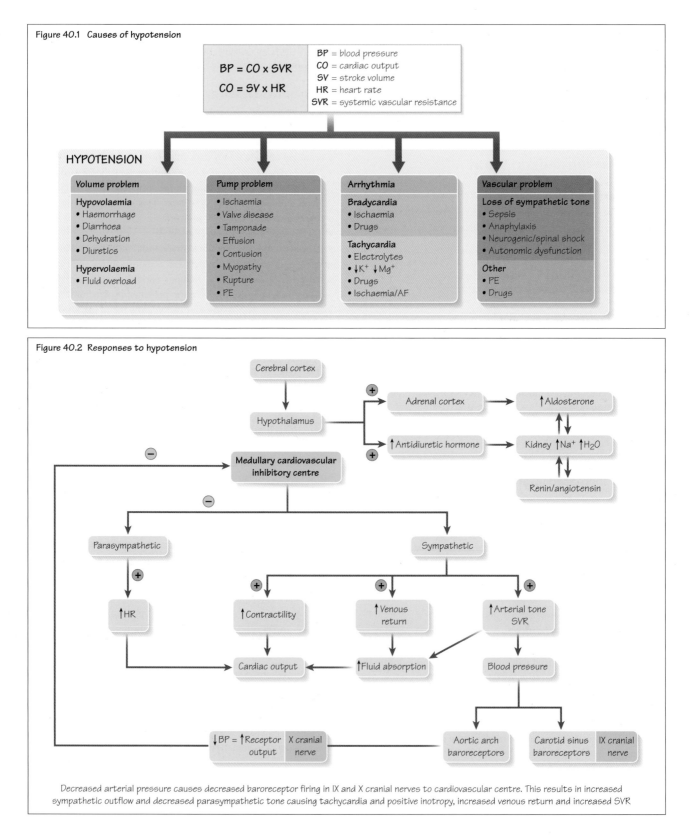

Figure 40.1 Causes of hypotension

BP = CO x SVR
CO = SV x HR

BP = blood pressure
CO = cardiac output
SV = stroke volume
HR = heart rate
SVR = systemic vascular resistance

HYPOTENSION

Volume problem

Hypovolaemia
• Haemorrhage
• Diarrhoea
• Dehydration
• Diuretics

Hypervolaemia
• Fluid overload

Pump problem
• Ischaemia
• Valve disease
• Tamponade
• Effusion
• Contusion
• Myopathy
• Rupture
• PE

Arrhythmia

Bradycardia
• Ischaemia
• Drugs

Tachycardia
• Electrolytes
• ↓K+ ↓Mg+
• Drugs
• Ischaemia/AF

Vascular problem

Loss of sympathetic tone
• Sepsis
• Anaphylaxis
• Neurogenic/spinal shock
• Autonomic dysfunction

Other
• PE
• Drugs

Figure 40.2 Responses to hypotension

Cerebral cortex

Hypothalamus

Adrenal cortex → ↑Aldosterone

↑Antidiuretic hormone → Kidney ↑Na+ ↑H2O

Renin/angiotensin

Medullary cardiovascular inhibitory centre

Parasympathetic

Sympathetic

↑HR

↑Contractility

↑Venous return

↑Arterial tone SVR

Cardiac output ← ↑Fluid absorption

Blood pressure

↓BP = ↑Receptor output | X cranial nerve

Aortic arch baroreceptors

Carotid sinus baroreceptors | IX cranial nerve

Decreased arterial pressure causes decreased baroreceptor firing in IX and X cranial nerves to cardiovascular centre. This results in increased sympathetic outflow and decreased parasympathetic tone causing tachycardia and positive inotropy, increased venous return and increased SVR

All patients have their 'obs' recorded at least once a day, so you **will** be asked about the significance of 'abnormal' blood pressure readings routinely. As hypotension can represent the first signs of a serious acute illness (Fig. 40.1) differentiating between a low 'normal' reading and an abnormal one is a vital skill. This chapter covers the assessment and management of patients with hypotension.

Definitions

Blood pressure

Blood pressure (BP) is defined as the force exerted by the blood per unit area of the vessel wall. Relating the mathematical to the physiological produces the equation:

BP = cardiac output (CO) × systemic vascular resistance (SVR)

This shows that to maintain an adequate BP you need an adequate flow of blood (CO) and adequate vascular tone (SVR). The flow from the heart (CO) is the volume of blood pumped each time the heart contracts per unit time (HR):

CO = stroke volume (SV) × heart rate (HR)

Hypotension

Hypotension is defined as a systolic BP of less than 90 mmHg or a diastolic BP less than 60 mmHg. There are many factors that influence blood pressure and pragmatically hypotension could be defined as a low blood pressure that causes symptoms or signs of inadequate organ perfusion (Fig. 40.2). Postural hypotension is an abnormal fall in BP of at least 20 mmHg systolic or 10 mmHg diastolic that occurs within 3 minutes of standing.

Symptoms and signs

- Dizziness/lightheadedness with or without a change of consciousness
- Weakness
- Fatigue
- Lethargy
- Sweating
- Visual disturbance
- Hearing disturbance
- Angina or palpitations (hypoperfusion of coronaries my aggravate angina or arrhythmias)
- Relation of symptoms to meals, urinary retention, constipation or erectile dysfunction with reduced sweating may suggest an autonomic cause

Causes

Considering the equations above, hypotension can be caused by a low CO or low SVR. A low CO can be caused by a low SV or a low HR. SV is determined by the filling, the stretch and the contractility of the muscle and the resistance to flow of the blood (SVR).

Acute hypotension

- Cardiogenic –
  - 'Pump failure' (e.g. ischaemia, contusion, myocarditis, myopathy, valvular or myocardial rupture)

  - Arrhythmia (i.e. too slow such that CO is low or too fast so that inadequate filling occurs affecting SV, or loss of atrial kick in atrial fibrillation (AF) reduces left ventricle (LV) filling by 30%)
- Hypovolaemic – inadequate intake compared to losses, e.g. bleeding, anaemia, dehydration, diarrhoea, diabetes mellitus and insipidus. A more profound effect occurs if the patient cannot mount a response, e.g spinal cord injury or underlying cardiac disease
- Obstructive – pulmonary embolism, atrial thrombus/tumour, tamponade, pneumothorax, constrictive pericarditis
- Distributive – sepsis, spinal shock, epidural/spinal anaesthesia

Chronic hypotension

- Autonomic dysfunction –
  - Central (e.g. motor neuron disease, multiple sclerosis, Parkinson's)
  - Peripheral (e.g. diabetes, Guillain–Barré, toxic neuropathies (alcohol, heavy metal poisoning), infectious neuropathies (Chagas, HIV related))
- Polypharmacy – antihypertensives, tricyclics, monoamine oxidase inhibitors, antiparkinsonian medications
- Endocrine/metabolic disorders – adrenocortical deficiency (Addison's), phaechromocytoma, electrolyte disturbances

Management

Treatment should be directed towards increasing SV or HR (by fluid filling, inotropes and chronotropes) or increasing SVR (vasoconstrictors).

Evaluate

- Is it genuine? Symptoms mean investigation or treatment. Measurement error (e.g. cuff size, placement)? History (trauma, postop, epidurals, new medications, otherwise stable)?
- Is HR appropriate? Too slow or too fast (low BP = ↑HR usually)
- What is volume status? Feel peripheries (cold = hypovolaemia, warm = distributive)
- Is the pump working? ECG, CXR, FBC, coags, U&Es, ABG

Acute hypotension

- Oxygen, airway support, IV access, fluids and inotropes
- Determine cause, start treatment and stop contributing medication

Chronic hypotension

- Fludrocortisone increases blood volume and enhances sensitivity of blood vessels to circulating catecholamines
- Stop contributing medications
- Recommend compression stockings
- Increased salt and water intake
- Consider endocrine (short synachthen test) and autonomic/tilt table testing

> **TOP TIPS**
>
> - Take hypotension seriously – assess the patient, especially if symptomatic and nursing colleagues are worried
> - Resuscitate (oxygen and fluids) while investigating the cause

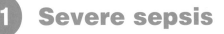

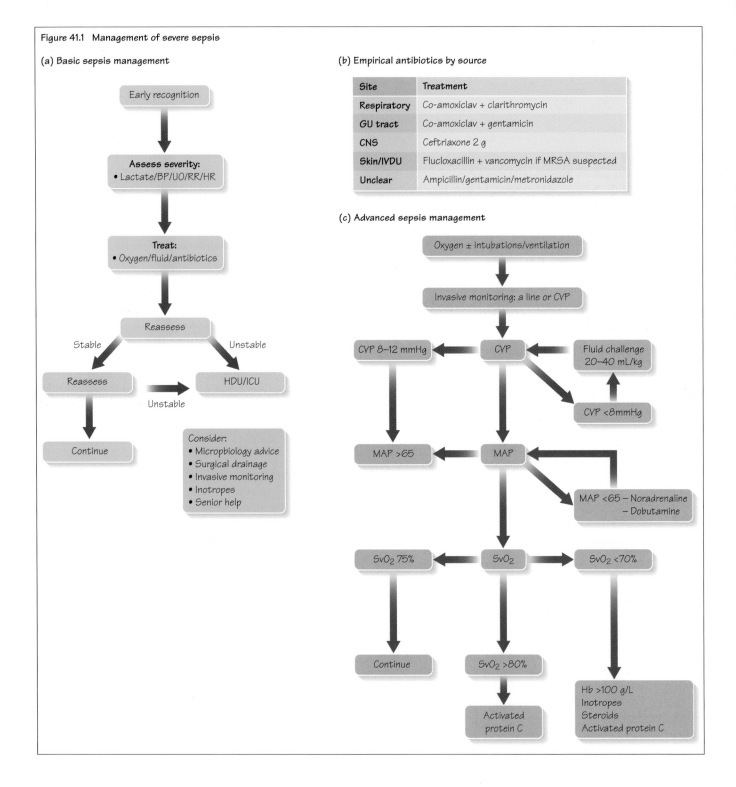

Figure 41.1 Management of severe sepsis

(a) Basic sepsis management

Early recognition

↓

Assess severity:
• Lactate/BP/UO/RR/HR

↓

Treat:
• Oxygen/fluid/antibiotics

↓

Reassess

Stable — Unstable

Reassess → HDU/ICU
Unstable

Continue

Consider:
• Micropbiology advice
• Surgical drainage
• Invasive monitoring
• Inotropes
• Senior help

(b) Empirical antibiotics by source

Site	Treatment
Respiratory	Co-amoxiclav + clarithromycin
GU tract	Co-amoxiclav + gentamicin
CNS	Ceftriaxone 2 g
Skin/IVDU	Flucloxacillin + vancomycin if MRSA suspected
Unclear	Ampicillin/gentamicin/metronidazole

(c) Advanced sepsis management

Oxygen ± intubations/ventilation

↓

Invasive monitoring: a line or CVP

↓

CVP 8–12 mmHg ← CVP ← Fluid challenge 20–40 mL/kg

CVP <8mmHg

MAP >65 ← MAP

MAP <65 – Noradrenaline – Dobutamine

SvO_2 75% ← SvO_2 → SvO_2 <70%

Continue SvO_2 >80%   Hb >100 g/L Inotropes Steroids Activated protein C

Activated protein C

 The Foundation Programme at a Glance, First Edition. Stuart Carney and Derek Gallen. © 2014 John Wiley & Sons, Ltd. Published 2014 by John Wiley & Sons, Ltd.

Sepsis from the Greek 'to putrify' occurs when a patient's response to a localized infection progresses to an uncontrolled systemic response. It can rapidly lead to multiorgan failure and death. After cardiovascular disease and stroke, it is the third most common cause of death in the UK, with a mortality rate of 35%. Early identification and treatment of sepsis saves lives This chapter covers the assessment and management of severe sepsis.

Definitions

Systemic inflammatory response syndrome (SIRS)

The response to inflammation produces a non-specific clinical response that has been described as SIRS. SIRS is defined as the presence of two or more of the following:

- Heart rate > 90 bpm
- Temperature < 36.0 or > 38.3°C
- Respiratory rate > 20 breaths per minute
- Acutely altered mental state
- Blood glucose > 7.7 mmol/L
- White cell count (WCC) < 4 or > 12 × 10^9/L

Sepsis

If there is a clinical suspicion of new infection in the context of SIRS then the patient has sepsis, e.g.:

- Respiratory – cough, sputum, chest pain
- Gastrointestinal – abdominal pain, distension, diarrhoea
- Cardiovascular – new murmurs, signs of endocarditis
- Gastrourinal – dysuria
- CNS – headache with neck stiffness
- Other – line infection, cellulitis, joint infection

Severe sepsis

If there is also evidence of organ dysfunction the patient has severe sepsis. Organ dysfunction may be manifest by:

- SPO_2 > 90% or SPO_2 > 94% on oxygen
- BP < 90 mmHg, systolic mean arterial pressure (MAP) < 65 mmHg after a fluid challenge
- Hyperbilirubinaemia
- Urine output < 0.5 mL/kg/h for 2 hours, creatinine > 177 μmol/L
- INR > 1.5 or activated partial thromboplastin time (APTT) > 60, platelets < 100 × 10^9 /L
- Lactate > 2 mmol/L after fluid resuscitation

Severe sepsis with hypotension that does not respond to fluid resuscitation (20–40 mL/kg bolus) is **septic shock**.

Incidence and risk factors

Severe sepsis is on the rise due to an increasingly elderly population, more patients who are immunocompromised, increased bacterial resistance and invasive surgery.

Risk factors include:

- Diabetes mellitus
- Trauma
- Burns
- Substance abuse
- Haematological disorders
- Recent surgery
- Indwelling catheters

Management

Treatment should be directed towards early antibiotics and source control, optimizing oxygen delivery, reducing oxygen demand and supporting appropriate physiological responses (Fig. 41.1). Management has been simplified into achievable care bundles, which can be delivered consistently to patients and prevent the progression of sepsis into severe sepsis and save lives. There is debate over certain aspects (steroids, activated protein C) of advanced treatment of severe sepsis.

Early management (1st hour)

The following should be achieved within 1 hour of sepsis being suspected:

- High-flow oxygen
- Blood cultures and microbiology samples as appropriate
- Source control
- Empirical IV antibiotics dependant on suspected source
- Fluid resuscitation
- Measurement of serum lactate
- Monitoring of urine output

Monitoring and reassessment (1–4 hours)

If the patient is responding to initial therapy it should be continued. Consider what level of further intervention may be required and by whom and where this can be delivered. Baseline investigations such as blood gases, CXR, ECG, U&Es, FBC as well as a full history and examination should be conducted.

The severity of illness should be assessed (persistent hypotension, lactate > 4 mmol/L, base deficit –5 to –10 mmol/L) and if unstable, early referral to 'critical care'.

Advanced management (1–6 hours)

Treatment can include:

- Intubation and ventilation
- Central venous pressure (CVP) monitoring: > 8 mmHg or > 12 mmHg if ventilated
- Measurement of mixed venous oxygen saturation:
  - SvO_2 75% – oxygen delivery adequate
  - SvO_2 < 70% – inadequate; consider intunbation, blood transfusion and noradrenaline to achieve MAP > 65 mmHg, and dobutamine to improve cardiac output
  - SvO_2 > 80% – inadequate oxygen utilization; consider activated protein C

TOP TIPS

- Resuscitate – oxygen, fluids
- Treat – early appropriate antibiotics and source control
- Reassess and relocate

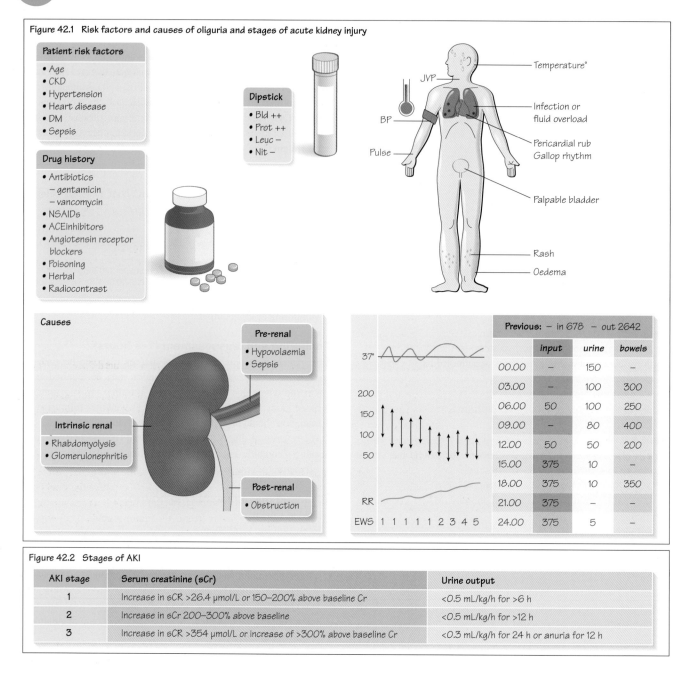

Figure 42.1   Risk factors and causes of oliguria and stages of acute kidney injury

Patient risk factors

- Age
- CKD
- Hypertension
- Heart disease
- DM
- Sepsis

Drug history

- Antibiotics
  - gentamicin
  - vancomycin
- NSAIDs
- ACEinhibitors
- Angiotensin receptor blockers
- Poisoning
- Herbal
- Radiocontrast

Dipstick

- Bld ++
- Prot ++
- Leuc –
- Nit –

Temperature°

JVP

BP

Pulse

Infection or fluid overload

Pericardial rub
Gallop rhythm

Palpable bladder

Rash

Oedema

Causes

Pre-renal
- Hypovolaemia
- Sepsis

Intrinsic renal
- Rhabdomyolysis
- Glomerulonephritis

Post-renal
- Obstruction

Previous: – in 678 – out 2642

	input	urine	bowels
00.00	–	150	–
03.00	–	100	300
06.00	50	100	250
09.00	–	80	400
12.00	50	50	200
15.00	375	10	–
18.00	375	10	350
21.00	375	–	–
24.00	375	5	–

37°

200
150
100
50

RR

EWS 1 1 1 1 1 2 3 4 5

Figure 42.2   Stages of AKI

AKI stage	Serum creatinine (sCr)	Urine output
1	Increase in sCR >26.4 µmol/L or 150–200% above baseline Cr	<0.5 mL/kg/h for >6 h
2	Increase in sCr 200–300% above baseline	<0.5 mL/kg/h for >12 h
3	Increase in sCR >354 µmol/L or increase of >300% above baseline Cr	<0.3 mL/kg/h for 24 h or anuria for 12 h

This chapter covers the general clinical approach to patients presenting with a reduction in urine output.

Oliguria and anuria are manifestations of acute kidney injury (AKI). Oliguria is defined as a urine output of < 400 mL per 24 hours in adults and anuria as a urine output of < 50 mL per 24 hours. Regardless of the underlying cause, AKI leads to a rapid reduction in glomerular filtration rate (GFR) over a period of hours to days. This leads to retention of nitrogenous waste products, metabolic disturbances and disordered fluid balance. AKI is defined in terms of its severity (Fig. 42.1).

It should be noted that the estimated GFR (eGFR) is not the same as the actual GFR and is not a reliable measure in AKI.

Presentation

Presentation can differ depending on the situation of the patient and the cause of the AKI. Sometimes, the cause of oliguria will be apparent (e.g. a patient with shock or acute urinary retention). A hospital inpatient often presents with a documented reduction in urine output whereas patients in the community may present with vague symptoms due to uraemia, and oliguria is observed subsequently. Patients in the community more commonly have a single renal insult whereas oliguria acquired in hospital is often multifactorial (e.g. a combination of cardiac dysfunction, diuretic use and sepsis). Prompt recognition and treatment of oliguria is essential to minimize the risk of severe AKI requiring renal replacement therapy.

It is important to distinguish between oliguria and anuria because the differential diagnosis of anuria is generally limited to total obstruction of the urinary tract, bilateral renovascular occlusion (or single kidney) or a severe necrotizing glomerulonephritis (like antiglomerular basement membrane disease).

For all patients with oliguria, you should consider whether the cause is likely to be pre-renal, renal or post-renal or a combination of these factors (e.g. hypovolaemia, hypotension, nephrotoxic drugs, sepsis, urinary tract obstruction). It is important to undertake a comprehensive history and examination as there are generally pointers to the cause in the history and examination

Prevention

Some patients are at particular risk of developing AKI (Fig. 42.1) so it is important to monitor BP, fluid balance and looking for signs of infection in these patients. Prompt recognition and treatment of oliguria can prevent AKI.

History

A full clinical history should be taken, including:
- Is the patient thirsty? (suggests volume depletion)
- Does the patient have a desire to void? (suggests obstruction)
- Any history suggestive of volume loss? (diarrhoea and/or vomiting, diuretics, GI blood loss, perioperative fluid losses, third-spacing)
- Any cardiac problems? (recent myocardial infarction (MI), heart failure, arrhythymias)
- Any infective symptoms? (fever, rigors, productive cough, abdominal pain/upset, dysuria)
- Any recent surgery, trauma or investigations? (blood loss, rhabdomyolysis, radioiodinated contrast used in CT scans and angiograms)
- Drug history? (ACE inhibitors, angiotensin-receptor blockers, diuretics, any new drugs, non-steroidal anti-inflammatory drug (NSAID) use – bear in mind many patients buy NSAIDs over the counter, so ask specifically about these)

Examination

A full clinical examination should be undertaken, including:
- Temperature
- Pulse rate and character
- Blood pressure – compared with the patient's baseline BP
- Jugular venous pressure (JVP)
- Heart sounds, e.g. cardiac murmur pericardial rub, gallop rhythm?
- Breath sounds – is there evidence of pulmonary oedema or infection?
- Is there a palpable bladder or other abdominal mass?
- Is the patient catheterized? If so, is the urine the colour of cola (rhadomyolysis) or is there significant haematuria (clot retention)?
- Is there any sacral or leg oedema?
- Have a general look for skin rashes or joint swelling
- **Look at patient's charts!** Look at BP trend, total input and output, temperature, early warning score (more general organ dysfunction?)

NB if the patient is catheterized, the catheter should be irrigated at this point to ensure patency before considering investigations.

Investigations

All patients should have the following:
- **FBC, clotting screen, U&E, venous bicarbonate, bone biochemistry, LFTs, glucose, CRP**
- **Blood cultures**
- Urine dipstick (and MSU unless dipstick is completely negative)

If the cause is apparent, investigations and management should be focused appropriately. Where no cause is immediately apparent, the following investigations should be considered:
- **Bladder scan** – useful ward test to look for urinary obstruction. If the patient has recently had a catheter removed and the bladder scan shows significant fluid volume, a further catheter may avoid the need for further (unnecessary) investigations
- **Ultrasound scan (USS)** – to exclude obstruction. All patients with AKI where there is no apparent volume depletion or catheter blockage should have an USS within 24 hours
- **Serum creatinine kinase (CK)** – if rhabdomyolysis is suspected (e.g. prolonged seizure, prolonged collapse on the floor)
- **Troponin I** – if a new cardiac event is suspected
- **ANA, C3/C4, ANCA, serum and urine electrophoresis** – if an intrinsic renal cause (glomerulonephritis) is possible (e.g. blood and/or protein on urine dipstick)
- **Antistreptolysin O (ASO) titres** – if postinfectious glomerulnephritis is suspected (recent upper respiratory infection). Uncommon

Management

Immediate management for all patients
- Stop ACE inhibitors, angiotensin receptor blockers and any other nephrotoxic drugs
- Assess fluid balance
- Treat infection promptly with appropriate antibiotics (discuss with microbiology)

If you suspect hypovolaemia ...
- Withhold all diuretics and antihypertensives until there is a clinical improvement
- Give a bolus of 500 mL of IV 0.9% saline (stat) and monitor the effect on pulse rate and BP. If there is an initial rise in BP and CVP but these quickly fall again, give a further 500 mL 0.9% saline fluid challenge and review again

Following further clinical examination it may be appropriate to administer a further slower intravenous fluid infusion. If there is a sustained rise in BP or you are unsure of the effect of the fluid bolus, the patient should be reviewed by a senior doctor. If a patient is elderly or has heart problems, the patient may require central line insertion.

If the patient has urinary obstruction ...
Relieve it! Place a urinary catheter. If the patient had hydronephrosis on USS a further USS will be necessary after a few days to demonstrate improvement. Refer to an urologist if urine output and serum creatinine do not improve or hydonephrosis on USS.

Ongoing management
- Discuss with a nephrologist if an intrinsic renal cause is suspected, or initial management does not improve urine output/renal function
- Optimize nutrition
- Review fluid balance frequently
- Consider restarting ACE inhibitor/angiotensin-receptor blocker when the patient has made a full clinical recovery

> **TOP TIPS**
>
> - Always take a drop in urine output seriously and immediately search for the underlying cause. Time is kidney (function)!
> - Always check for a blockage to urine output in anuria
> - Look at fluid balance carefully and remember to consider things not always charted like vomiting and diarrhoea in your assessment
> - Stop any nephrotoxic drugs in patients with anuria
> - Avoid giving radiocontrast to patients with reduced urine output/AKI

Figure 43.1 Causes of hyperkalaemia

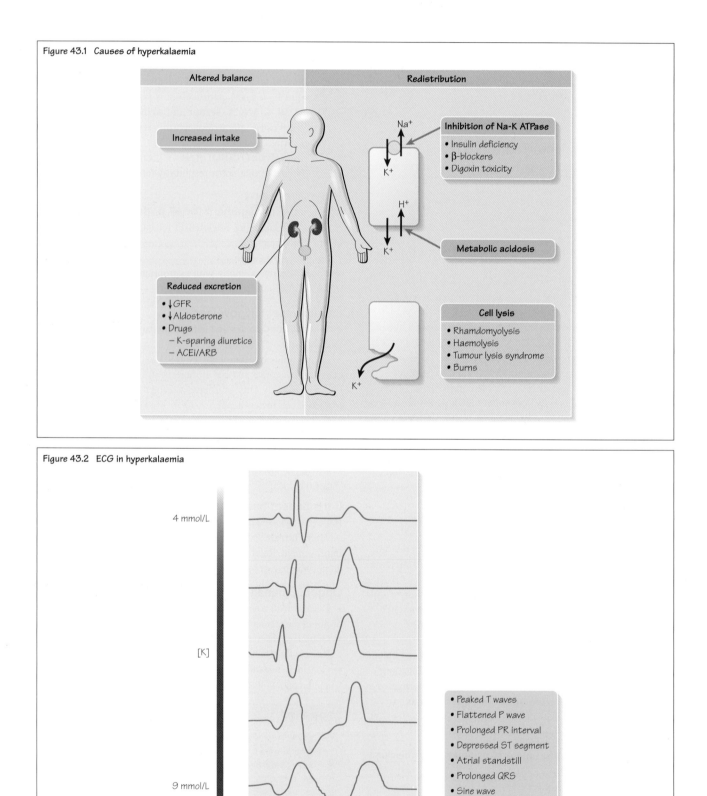

Altered balance	Redistribution

Increased intake

Inhibition of Na-K ATPase
- Insulin deficiency
- β-blockers
- Digoxin toxicity

Na⁺

K⁺

H⁺

K⁺

Metabolic acidosis

Reduced excretion
- ↓GFR
- ↓Aldosterone
- Drugs
  - K-sparing diuretics
  - ACEi/ARB

Cell lysis
- Rhamdomyolysis
- Haemolysis
- Tumour lysis syndrome
- Burns

K⁺

Figure 43.2 ECG in hyperkalaemia

4 mmol/L

[K]

9 mmol/L

- Peaked T waves
- Flattened P wave
- Prolonged PR interval
- Depressed ST segment
- Atrial standstill
- Prolonged QRS
- Sine wave
- Asystole

This chapter and Chapter 44 cover the pathophysiology, diagnosis and management of patients with the two most common and potentially dangerous electrolyte disturbances – hyperkalaemia and hyponatraemia.

Electrolyte derangements can effect up to 22% of hospitalized patients. Common clinically significant electrolyte derangements include hyperkalaemia and hyponatraemia.

Hyperkalaemia

The intracellular/extracellular K^+ ratio is the major determinant of the resting membrane potential. Minor changes in the extracellular potassium concentration can have a dramatic impact on the function of excitable tissues such as the heart and neuromuscular cells. Hyperkalaemia is therefore a medical emergency that demands immediate attention.

Under normal circumstances the excretory capacity of the kidney is so great that hyperkalaemia is unusual in the absence of renal impairment (GFR < 20 mL/min). In hyperkalaemic patients with preserved renal function, a defect in aldosterone activity needs to be considered.

Presentation
- Often asymptomatic – detected by measurement of the serum electrolytes
- Symptomatic – may present with muscle weakness, ascending paralysis, paraesthesia and, in severe cases, with respiratory compromise, cardiac arrest and sudden death. Symptoms related to the underlying cause of the hyperkalaemia may be present (Fig. 43.1)

History
A full history should be taken, particularly asking about:
- Recent drug use, particularly K^+-sparing diuretics, ACE inhibitors and angiotensin receptor blockers, β-blockers and NSAIDs
- Past medical history of chronic kidney disease, adrenal disease (e.g. Addison's disease) and diabetes mellitus
- Symptoms suggestive of acute kidney injury (oliguria, oedema)
- Symptoms of potential causes of AKI (acute volume loss (diarrhoea/vomiting, acute blood loss), heart failure, urinary obstruction)
- Muscle injury, recent chemotherapy and acute haemolysis
- Intake of a potassium load (potassium-rich diet, salt substitutes (contain KCl), blood transfusion)

Examination
The examination should look for:
- Evidence of a pre-renal state or urinary tract obstruction causing acute kidney injury
- Blood pressure
- Evidence of muscle injury
- Features of adrenal insufficiency
- Neuromuscular deficit

Investigations
Hyperkalaemia is a medical emergency and initial investigations should be directed at the consequences of hyperkalaemia. The cause can be investigated once the patient's potassium level is safe.

Investigations to seek the consequences of hyperkalaemia
- ECG – evidence of hyperkalaemia-induced conduction abnormalities (Fig. 43.1) indicates a need for urgent treatment

Investigations to seek the causes of hyperkalaemia
- Serum urea and electrolytes to assess renal function

- Arterial blood gases to assess acid–base status
- Serum creatine kinase, phosphate and urate if rhabdomyolysis or tumour lysis syndrome is suspected
- Renin, aldosterone and cortisol levels if adrenal insufficiency is suspected

Management
Hyperkalaemia is classified as mild (K^+ 5.5–6.0 mmol/L), moderate (K^+ 6.1–6.5 mmol/L) or severe (K^+ > 6.5 mmol/L or if any K^+-associated ECG changes or muscle symptoms).

Eliminate the underlying cause, e.g. stop potassium-containing medications.

Severe hyperkalaemia
This requires urgent treatment. Continuous cardiac monitoring should be instituted.
1 Actions to antagonize the cell membrane actions of hyperkalaemia:
- Intravenous calcium: inject 10 mL of 10% calcium chloride or gluconate over 2–3 minutes
- ECG should normalize in 1–3 minutes. The effect is transient and the dose can be repeated
- Note that the K^+ concentration is unaffected
2 Actions to increase K^+ entry into cells (using one or a combination of the treatments below):
- Soluble insulin (10 units) with 50% dextrose in water solution (50 mL) over 1 hour. Can be repeated if necessary. Monitor blood glucose carefully!
- High-dose $β_2$-adrenergic agonist (salbutamol) as IV injection (0.5 mg) or nebulized inhaler (10–20 mg)
- Intravenous sodium bicarbonate (50–100 mmol) in patients with metabolic acidosis
3 Actions to eliminate excess potassium from the body:
- Volume expansion with normal saline followed by IV furosemide/frusemide once volume replete. This is only useful in patients with pre-renal AKI due to volume depletion
- Resin exchanger (e.g. calcium resonium) given either orally or as a retention enema
- Dialysis for patients with advanced renal failure in whom other measures are unsuccessful

Mild hyperkalaemia
This can usually be managed by eliminating the underlying cause (e.g. discontinuing K^+-sparing diuretics) and restricting dietary potassium intake.

Moderate hyperkalaemia
Additional measures such as loop diuretics, synthetic mineralocorticoids and exchange resins can be considered.

TOP TIPS

- Do an ECG immediately in anyone with hyperkalaemia
- Give intravenous calcium immediately if the ECG shows hyperkalaemic changes
- If the GFR is over 20 mL/min, consider a defect of the rennin/angiotensin/aldosterone pathway
- Inform the renal team early if a hyperkalaemic patient has significant renal impairment – dialysis is likely to be necessary

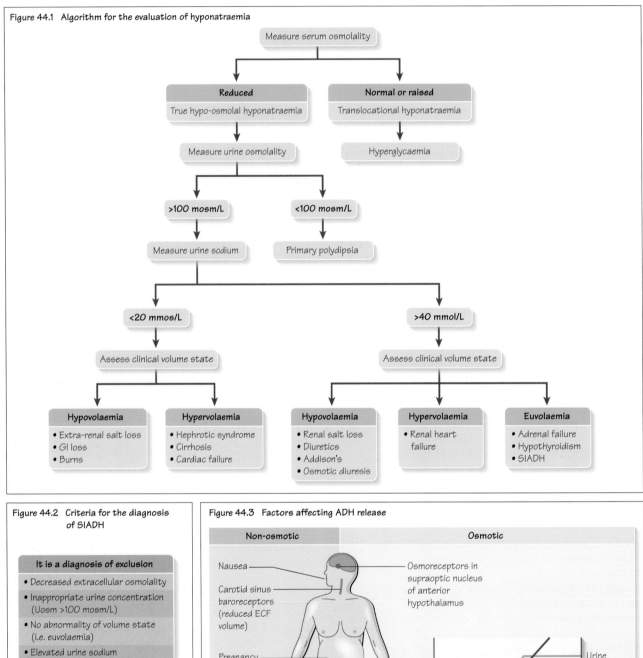

Figure 44.1 Algorithm for the evaluation of hyponatraemia

Measure serum osmolality

Reduced	Normal or raised
True hypo-osmolal hyponatraemia	Translocational hyponatraemia

Measure urine osmolality → Hyperglycaemia

>100 mosm/L → Measure urine sodium

<100 mosm/L → Primary polydipsia

<20 mmos/L → Assess clinical volume state

>40 mmol/L → Assess clinical volume state

Hypovolaemia
- Extra-renal salt loss
- GI loss
- Burns

Hypervolaemia
- Hephrotic syndrome
- Cirrhosis
- Cardiac failure

Hypovolaemia
- Renal salt loss
- Diuretics
- Addison's
- Osmotic diuresis

Hypervolaemia
- Renal heart failure

Euvolaemia
- Adrenal failure
- Hypothyroidism
- SIADH

Figure 44.2 Criteria for the diagnosis of SIADH

It is a diagnosis of exclusion
- Decreased extracellular osmolality
- Inappropriate urine concentration (Uosm >100 mosm/L)
- No abnormality of volume state (i.e. euvolaemia)
- Elevated urine sodium concentration (>40 mmol/L)
- No adrenal, renal, thyroid, pituitary disease
- No diuretic use

Figure 44.3 Factors affecting ADH release

Non-osmotic	Osmotic

Nausea

Carotid sinus baroreceptors (reduced ECF volume)

Pregnancy

Pain

Osmoreceptors in supraoptic nucleus of anterior hypothalamus

Plasma ADH concentration

Urine osmolarity

280   290

Serum osmolality (mosm/L)

This chapter and Chapter 43 cover the pathophysiology, diagnosis and management of patients with the two most common and potentially dangerous electrolyte disturbances – hyperkalaemia and hyponatraemia.

Electrolyte derangements can effect up to 22% of hospitalized patients. Common clinically significant electrolyte derangements include hyperkalaemia and hyponatraemia.

Hyponatraemia

The serum sodium concentration is the main determinant of extracellular osmolality. Therefore, hyponatraemia results in a reduction in extracellular osmolality and generates an osmotic gradient that favours the movement of water into cells. The major consequence of this is brain swelling within the confines of the cranium, which leads to increased intracranial pressure.

Regulation of osmolality requires an intact thirst mechanism, regulated antidiuretic hormone (ADH) secretion, and normal renal function. Hyponatraemia usually results from defective urinary dilution (usually due to ADH secretion) and ongoing water ingestion. In hyponatraemic patients the main question to address is why ADH secretion is not suppressed in the face of reduced osmolality.

The factors that induce ADH secretion are indicated in Fig. 44.1. In hyponatraemic patients the non-osmotic factors are often key.

It is also important to recognize that hyponatraemia can occur in the presence of *increased* extracellular osmolality (translocational hyponatraemia). This is usually caused by hyperglycaemia, which generates an osmotic gradient that pulls water out of cells. This results in dilution of the extracellular sodium (hyponatraemia) and cell shrinkage rather than swelling. The clinical consequences are therefore very different.

Presentation

Hyponatraemia may be asymptomatic or associated with symptoms caused by brain swelling. The severity of symptoms depends on the rapidity of onset of hyponatraemia and the magnitude of reduction of serum sodium. Typical symptoms include anorexia, malaise, nausea, vomiting, headache, lethargy, confusion, seizures, coma and, if untreated, brain herniation, respiratory arrest and death. Severe symptoms are more common in children, menstruating females, hypoxic patients and patients with brain injury.

History

Patients should be asked about:
- Fluid intake
- Past medical history of malignant disease, thyroid or adrenal disease, heart disease, psychiatric disease
- Recent drug use, particularly diuretics and antidepressants
- Symptoms of volume depletion or volume overload
- Symptoms related to brain oedema

Examination

The most important aspect of the examination is an accurate assessment of the volume state. An accurate neurological examination should also be undertaken (including fundoscopy).

Investigations

All patients should have the following:
- Serum electrolytes and osmolality
- Blood glucose
- Urine osmolality and sodium concentration
- Thyroid and adrenal (and possibly pituitary) function tests in selected cases

An algorithm for the evaluation of the cause of hyponatraemia is shown at the top of Fig. 44.1, and the diagnostic criteria for the syndrome of inappropirate ADH (SIADH) are shown in Fig. 44.2.

Management

Morbidity and mortality are related to neurological complications of either acute cerebral oedema in severe, acute cases or central pontine myelinolysis (CPM) due to inappropriate management (too rapid correction or overcorrection) in more chronic cases.

Treatment choices depend on the severity of the symptoms, the rapidity of onset of hyponatraemia and the patient's volume state.
- *Acute and symptomatic hyponatraemia* requires prompt treatment. Failure to do so risks further brain oedema, tentorial herniation and death. Senior help should be sought immediately. Treatment involves administration of hypertonic (3%) saline with IV furosemide/frusemide to enhance free-water excretion. The treatment aim is to increase serum sodium concentration by 1–2 mmol/L/h until symptoms resolve (usually serum sodium 120–125 mmol/L)
- *Chronic, symptomatic hyponatraemia* requires cautious treatment. Overaggressive correction risks CPM. The rate of correction should not exceed 1 mmol/L/h
- *Asymptomatic hyponatraemia* can usually be managed by focusing on the underlying cause. In euvolaemic patients the mainstay of treatment is restriction of fluid intake, usually to < 1 L/day. Supplementation of the diet with salt or protein may also be helpful. Vasopressin receptor antagonists have recently been licensed although their clinical role is still under evaluation

---

TOP TIPS

- An understanding of basic physiology of water reguialation helps with the evaluation of patients with hyponatraemia
- Treat symptomatic hyponatraemia as a medical emergency
- Don't delay getting senior support
- Assessment of the patient's volume state is key to identifying the cause of hyponatraemia
- Asymptomatic hyponatraemic patients should be corrected very slowly to avoid brainstem demyelination

45 Diabetic ketoacidosis

Figure 45.1 Management guideline for diabetic ketoacidosis

Immediate assessment and management. 0 to 60 minutes

Recognition/diagnosis
- Ill patient, reduced GCS
- Polyuria, dehydration – tachycardia, hypotension
- Acidosis – tachypnoea, low pH and bicarbonate
- Hyperglycaemia
- Ketonaemia or ketones in urine (+2 or greater)
- Aetiology – missed insulin, illness or infection, new case

Assess. Severe if any present of...
- SBP <90 mmHg
- Pulse <60 or >100 bpm
- GCS <12
- O₂ sats <92% on air
- Plasma ketones >6 mmol/L
- Venous/arterial pH <7.1 or bicarbonate <5 mmol/L
- Hypokalaemia <3.5 mmol/L

Aims
- Think ABC to stabilize the patient
- Ensure oxygenation, restore circulation, begin to correct acidosis and electrolytes
- Reduce harm – level 2 or HDU nursing
- Keep NBM
- Place NG tube if GCS <12, consider thromboprophylaxis
- Seek and treat cause of DKA
- Review and ensure your familiarity with hospital DKA management guideline

Immediate actions
- In severe cases, call for senior help
- Insert large bore cannula, transfer to HDU
- Commence IV N saline and insulin infusions (see boxes)
- Establish hourly monitoring of pulse, BP, O₂ sats, respiratory rate, GCS, capillary glucose
- Complete clinical, biochemical and radiological assessment
- Contact diabetes team as soon as possible

Fluid regimen
- Commence N saline 1000 mL over 1 h, unless... systolic BP <90 mmHg – give 500 mL N saline in 15 min **whilst awaiting senior input**
- If systolic remains <90 mmHg repeat 500 mL N saline in 15 min and **call for immediate senior assistance**
- At 1 h or if systolic BP >90 mmHg give...
  1000 mL N saline in 1 h, then
  1000 mL N saline with KCl over 2 h
  1000 mL N saline with KCl over 2 h
  1000 mL N saline with KCl over 4 h
  1000 mL N saline with KCl over 4 h
- Caution in young 18–25, elderly >60, pregnancy, cardiac, renal disease or other co-morbidity

Reassess hydration requirements at 12 hours

Establish fixed rate insulin infusion
- Obtain or estimate patient's body weight
- Prepare human soluble insulin 50 units in 50 mL N saline
- Connect insulin via fluids cannula using a one-way valve
- Infuse at 0.1 unit/kg/h (e.g. 7 mL/h if weight is 70 kg)
- Give stat dose 0.1 unit/kg IM if infusion start delayed
- Continue normal long-acting insulin at usual dose & time

Potassium replacement
>5.5 mmol/L	Nil. Continue to monitor plasma levels	
3.5–5.5 mmol/L	40 mmol KCl in each 1000 mL N saline (faster rates are unsafe by peripheral ivi)	
<3.5 mmol/L	**Senior review needed.** Patient may require potassium infusion via central line	

1 hour to 12 hours

Aims
- Continue to suppress ketogenesis with insulin
- Lower ketones in plasma to <0.3 mmol/L
- Raise venous bicarbonate to >18 mmol/L
- Lower plasma glucose to around 14 mmol/L
- Maintain potassium >3.5 to <5.5 mmol/L

Observation and measurements
- Monitor fluid balance. Consider urinary catheter
- Monitor vital signs. Complete EW scoring inc O₂ sats
- Measure plasma ketones and glucose hourly
- Measure venous pH, bicarbonate, glucose and potassium at 60 min, 2 and 4 h (or more frequently if required)

Treatments
- Continue fluid replacement with potassium as indicated above
- Continue fixed rate insulin at 0.1 unit/kg/h until blood ketones <0.3 mmol/L, venous pH >7.3 and/or venous bicarbonate >18 mmol/L. **Call for senior review again if the biochemical parameters are not improving**

If plasma glucose falls to <14 mmol/L give 10% dextrose solution 125 mL/h in addition to N saline infusion

Resolution

Resolution phase. Continue IV regimen until...
- Patient eating and drinking, vital signs normal and biochemistry normalized as indicated above
- Then restart normal fast-acting insulin with meals and discontinue the IV insulin 60 min later
- Continue to treat predisposing causes

Based on Joint British Diabetes Societies publication, March 2010

This chapter covers the recognition, causes and immediate management of diabetic ketoacidosis (DKA) and highlights the commonest causes of death during DKA.

Recognition and management of DKA

DKA is diagnosed by the presence of the biochemical triad of metabolic acidosis, ketonaemia and hyperglycaemia. It is the commonest serious complication of type 1 diabetes. DKA has high mortality and morbidity but much of this is preventable by early recognition and good-quality clinical management.

It is often junior members of the medical team who first encounter a patient with DKA, so understanding of the metabolic derangement and its immediate management are mandatory for all foundation doctors.

Most hospitals have their own guideline for management of DKA. These often vary and may be out of date. This chapter summarizes current best practice in the management of DKA as agreed by the Joint British Diabetes Societies in March 2010 (Fig. 45.1).

Pathophysiology

Absolute or relative insulin deficiency prevents cellular glucose uptake, permits uncontrolled gluconeogenesis and glycogenolysis raising plasma glucose, and allows uncontrolled lipolysis producing free fatty acids and triglycerides. As the patient becomes unwell, insulin counterregulatory hormones cortisol, growth hormone and glucagon are released, compounding these changes.

Intracellular glucose deficiency prevents normal aerobic metabolism. Cells switch to free fatty acids as an alternative fuel, liberating ketoacids. Vomiting due to acidosis along with an osmotic diuresis due to hyperglycaemia causes dehydration, circulatory collapse and poor tissue perfusion, compounding the acidosis. Sick cells leak potassium, raising plasma potassium which is then excreted in the urine, resulting in low total body potassium.

Aetiology

- **Absolute insulin deficiency** (50% of cases) is caused by:
  - Failure to inject
  - Failure of insulin delivery devices or pumps
  - New diagnosis of type 1 diabetes
- **Relative insulin deficiency** results from a failure to increase insulin doses during illness. It occurs when type 1 patients:
  - Are physically stressed by illness, often infection
  - Suffer trauma, surgery, etc.

Counterregulatory hormone release **increases insulin requirements even if patients are unable to eat**. Failure to match insulin requirement results in DKA.

Mortality and morbidity

With best care mortality remains around 1%. With poor-quality care it is around 8%. Severe hypokalaemia is the commonest cause of death, followed by cerebral oedema especially in children and young adults, then aspiration pneumonia and respiratory distress syndrome (RDS).

Treatment

Rationale for best practice

The absolute deficiencies in DKA are of insulin, water, sodium and potassium. Correct these appropriately and the metabolic derangement will resolve.

1 **Commence infusion of N saline**. Immediate fluid resuscitation (Fig 45.1) improves tissue perfusion, cardiac function and tissue oxygen delivery.

2 **Commence fixed rate insulin infusion**. High-dose (0.1 unit/kg/h) insulin turns off lipolysis, gluconeogenesis and glycogenolysis. It drives glucose into cells where it can now be used for aerobic metabolism. Continue the patient's usual long-acting insulin.

3 **Replace potassium from 1 hour**. With fluid, oxygen, insulin and intracellular glucose, sick cells recover and potassium re-uptake into cells occurs, lowering plasma potassium very rapidly.

4 **Provide substrate when capillary glucose is < 14 mol/L**. The metabolic derangement of DKA has not been corrected until ketonaemia is eliminated. Continued high-dose insulin infusion is needed to achieve this. Many type 1 diabetic patients now respond to illness by increasing their insulin doses and will have partially treated their own hyperglycaemia before admission. As a result it becomes necessary to provide additional glucose substrate as a 10% dextrose infusion, 125 mL/h, alongside continued fluid resuscitation with saline. 'Sliding scale' insulin regimens permit low-dose insulin delivery and **are no longer recommended**.

Patient care

Even best metabolic management can be undone by poor-quality nursing and monitoring, or failure to identify and adequately treat predisposing causes of DKA. Thus:

- Severe DKA needs level 2 (high dependency unit (HDU)) nursing care
- Monitor and respond to rising early warning scores (EWS)
- Nastogastric (NG) tube for obtunded or vomiting patients
- Consider need for thromboprophylaxis
- Measure capillary glucose and ketones hourly with venous plasma bicarbonate and pH
- Arterial bloods are **not required** if the patient is not hypoxaemic (if O_2 sats > 92% on air)
- Refer to the diabetes team as soon as possible

Resolution phase

When the patient is eating and drinking, plasma ketones < 0.3 mmol/L, pH > 7.3 and/or venous bicarbonate > 18 mmol/L restart patient's normal fast-acting insulin doses and discontinue the IV regimen 60 minutes later.

TOP TIPS

- DKA can be caused by absolute or relative insulin deficiency
- Stress hormones (cortisol, adrenaline, glucagon, growth hormone) cause insulin requirements to be high in poorly patients, even if they are not eating
- Treatment of DKA involves giving insulin, IV fluids and potassium plus treatment of the causative illness
- Early involvement of the specialist diabetes team is mandatory

Figure 46.1 Hypoglycaemia assessment and treatment

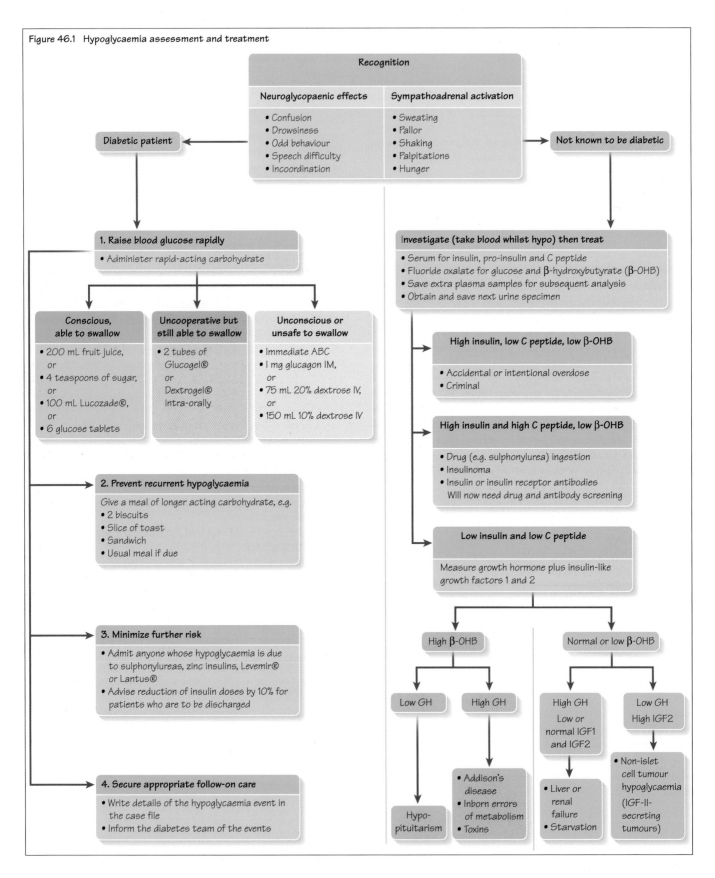

The Foundation Programme at a Glance, First Edition. Stuart Carney and Derek Gallen. © 2014 John Wiley & Sons, Ltd. Published 2014 by John Wiley & Sons, Ltd.

This chapter covers the recognition and management of hypoglycaemia in patients with diabetes and the biochemical investigation of hypoglycaemia in those not known to have diabetes (Fig. 46.1).

Hypoglycaemia is a medical emergency. If not recognized, investigated and treated with utmost urgency it can cause neurological damage, accidental physical injury or both. Hypoglycaemia in adults is most commonly due to excess insulin or sulphonylurea ingestion. However, it can also occur as a manifestation of other disease processes – diagnosis and treatment of which can abolish the hypoglycaemic episodes.

Recognition of hypoglycaemia

Clinical manifestations of hypoglycaemia (Fig. 46.1) occur when plasma glucose is < 3 mmol/L. It should be suspected in any acutely unwell, uncooperative or drowsy diabetic patient. Neuroglycopaenic symptoms result from cerebral glucose deprivation and autonomic symptoms occur as a result of counterregulatory sympathetic system activation and catecholamine release.

Spontaneous hypoglycaemia

Spontaneous hypoglycaemia in non-diabetics is rare but must be considered in any patient with episodic symptoms compatible with hypoglycaemia, loss of consciousness or seizures. In such patients timely collection (during hypoglycaemia) of samples for later assay is crucial to reach the correct diagnosis (Fig. 46.1).

Causes of hypoglycaemia in diabetes

Hypoglycaemia in diabetes is mild if it can be self-treated and severe if third party assistance is required.

Hypoglycaemia can occur in diabetic patients treated with insulin, sulphonylureas or meglitinides. Metformin, thiazolidinediones, DPP-4 inhibitors and GLP-1 analogues do not cause hypoglycaemia unless used in addition to insulin or sulphonylureas.

In hypoglycaemic diabetic patients consider:
- Insulin dosing or prescription errors (e.g. 4 units can be misread as 40 units)
- Patient on a 'nil by mouth' order
- Recent use of additional doses of short-acting insulin to correct hyperglycaemia
- IV insulin with no concomitant glucose infusion
- Missed meals or snacks
- Vomiting, poor appetite, poor oral hygiene
- Poor injection technique and/or abnormal injection sites
- Recovery from acute illness
- Cessation of high-dose glucocorticoids
- β-blockers (limit counterregulatory response and blunt sympathetic warning symptoms)

Risk factors for hypoglycaemia in diabetes

A patient's risk of hypoglycaemia is increased by:
1 **Lifestyle factors:**
  - Erratic lifestyle and glucose monitoring
  - Unaccustomed exercise
  - Increasing age
  - Alcohol consumption
2 **Clinical associations:**
  - Very tight glucose control
  - Recent severe hypoglycaemia
  - Unrecognized nocturnal hypoglycaemia
  - Long duration diabetes
  - Recent delivery and/or breastfeeding
  - Malabsorption or vomiting
  - Renal or liver failure
  - Metastatic carcinoma

Treatment

Provide rapid-acting carbohydrates to raise blood glucose followed by long-acting carbohydrate to maintain normal glucose levels (Fig. 46.1).

Rapid-acting carbohydrates include 200 mL pure fruit juice or 4 heaped teaspoons of sugar dissolved in water. Alternatively use 100 mL of Lucozade® or 6 dextrose tablets. A confused patient who is still able to swallow can be treated with 2 tubes of either Glucogel® or Dextrogel® squeezed into the buccal or oral cavity.

Unconscious patients need either glucagon 1 mg IM (can take 15 minutes to raise blood glucose and less effective after sulphonylureas), 75 mL of 20% or 150 mL of 10% dextrose IV over 10 minutes (50% dextrose is no longer recommended due to risk of extravasation injury). A fitting patient is best treated with IV dextrose if venous access is possible, due to its more rapid onset of action.

Once the patient has recovered it is essential to give a larger portion of longer acting carbohydrate such as two biscuits, a slice of toast, a glass of milk or a usual meal (as long as it contains carbohydrate). Failure to achieve this can result in a further episode of hypoglycaemia.

Follow on care

Diabetic patients who have recovered from hypoglycaemia may be allowed to go home unless:
- Treated with sulphonylureas or meglitinides
- On long-acting zinc insulins, insulin determir (Levemir®) or glargine (Lantus®)

Do not omit an insulin injection if one is due, but recommend to the patient that they reduce their dose by 10% until review by their diabetes team.

Document the episode and treatment in the case notes.

Always inform the diabetes team that a patient has suffered a hypoglycaemic episode. They will usually wish to review the patient as a matter of urgency.

TOP TIPS

- Hypoglycaemia causes symptoms of both neuroglycopaenia and sympathoadrenal activation
- In patients with diabetes, blood glucose must be raised rapidly before thinking about causation and prevention of recurrent episodes
- In patients without diabetes, immediate blood samples taken during hypoglycaemia are crucial to diagnosis

Figure 47.1 Types and causes of abdominal pain

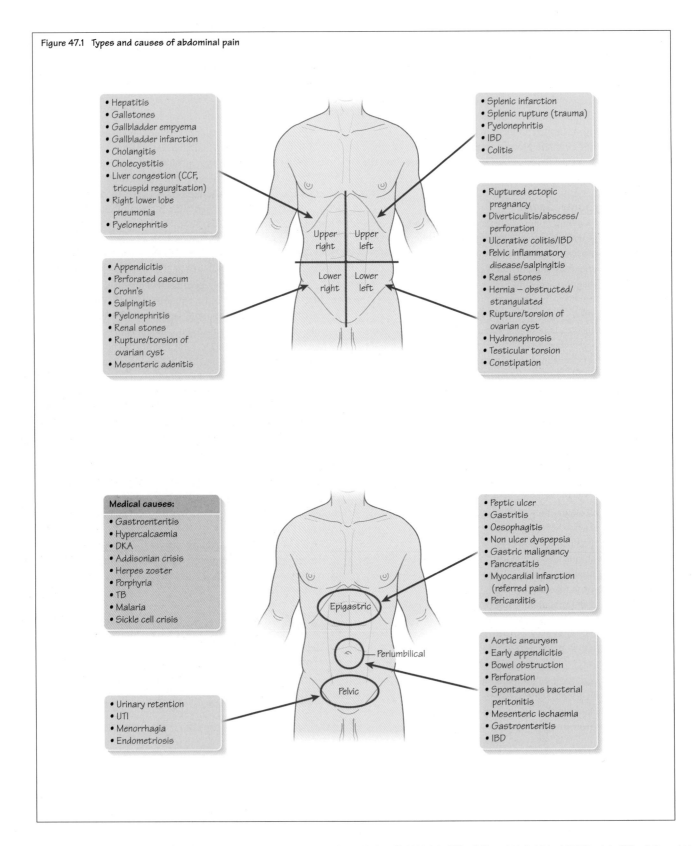

- Hepatitis
- Gallstones
- Gallbladder empyema
- Gallbladder infarction
- Cholangitis
- Cholecystitis
- Liver congestion (CCF, tricuspid regurgitation)
- Right lower lobe pneumonia
- Pyelonephritis

- Splenic infarction
- Splenic rupture (trauma)
- Pyelonephritis
- IBD
- Colitis

- Ruptured ectopic pregnancy
- Diverticulitis/abscess/perforation
- Ulcerative colitis/IBD
- Pelvic inflammatory disease/salpingitis
- Renal stones
- Hernia – obstructed/strangulated
- Rupture/torsion of ovarian cyst
- Hydronephrosis
- Testicular torsion
- Constipation

- Appendicitis
- Perforated caecum
- Crohn's
- Salpingitis
- Pyelonephritis
- Renal stones
- Rupture/torsion of ovarian cyst
- Mesenteric adenitis

Upper right   Upper left
Lower right   Lower left

Medical causes:
- Gastroenteritis
- Hypercalcaemia
- DKA
- Addisonian crisis
- Herpes zoster
- Porphyria
- TB
- Malaria
- Sickle cell crisis

- Peptic ulcer
- Gastritis
- Oesophagitis
- Non ulcer dyspepsia
- Gastric malignancy
- Pancreatitis
- Myocardial infarction (referred pain)
- Pericarditis

Epigastric

Periumbilical

Pelvic

- Aortic aneurysm
- Early appendicitis
- Bowel obstruction
- Perforation
- Spontaneous bacterial peritonitis
- Mesenteric ischaemia
- Gastroenteritis
- IBD

- Urinary retention
- UTI
- Menorrhagia
- Endometriosis

 The Foundation Programme at a Glance, First Edition. Stuart Carney and Derek Gallen. © 2014 John Wiley & Sons, Ltd. Published 2014 by John Wiley & Sons, Ltd.

This chapter covers the assessment of a patient with abdominal pain and the common causes. There are many causes of abdominal pain (Fig. 47.1), it is a very common presenting complaint. A clear history, focused examination and key investigations help to differentiate the underlying diagnosis. It is vital to identify those conditions that require urgent intervention (the acute abdomen).

History

- Site – where is it? Has it changed over time? Any radiation?
- Quality – what is it like? Sharp/dull/burning? Constant/colicky?
- Intensity – how severe is the pain? Does the intensity vary?
- Timing – speed of onset? Sudden/gradual? Duration (minutes/hours/weeks)? Relationship to eating, bowels, breathing, moving, micturition and periods? Frequency?
- Associated features – diarrhoea/vomiting/per rectum (PR) bleeding/melaena/back pain/jaundice/urinary symptoms/sweating/dizziness/fevers?
- Aggravating/relieving factors?
- Prior episodes
- Past medical history – any medical conditions causing recurrent abdominal pain? Crohn's? Gallstones? Hypertension? Ischaemic heart disease? AF?
- Past surgical history – prior operations leading to adhesions and obstruction? Is there a history of a known aneurysm?
- Possibility of pregnancy – think ectopic pregnancy in any female of child-bearing age
- Has there been any trauma? Think splenic rupture

Examination

- General – pain at rest? Anaemia? Jaundice? Lymphadenopathy? Any extraintestinal features to suggest inflammatory bowel disease?
- Observations – temperature (sepsis). Heart rate/BP/respiratory rate – markers of shock. Saturations. Capillary refill time (shock)
- Abdominal examination
- Inspection – scars, masses, jaundice, pain, distension (?obstruction), hernias, discolouration, bruising
- Palpation – presence of guarding/rebound tenderness suggesting peritonism? Are there any masses present? Presence of organomegaly? Is there a palpable abdominal aortic aneurysm (AAA)? Hernia – tender, reducible? Murphy's sign (cholecysitis)?
- Percussion – tympanic – signalling obstruction, enlarged bladder suggesting urinary retention, organomegaly, shifting dullness of ascites
- Auscultation – bowel sounds – may be absent in acute abdomen. Tinkling bowel sounds in obstruction
- Hernial orifices – any evidence of incarcerated hernia?
- Rectal examination (PR bleeding)
- Vaginal/testicular examination as appropriate

Investigations

All patients should have FBC (Hb drop in AAA/peptic ulcer) C-reactive protein (CRP)/erythrocyte sedimentation rate (ESR) (infection, abscess, irritable bowel disease (IBD)), U&E (renal failure), LFTs (gallstones, cholecytitis, cholangitis), bone (hypercalcaemia, renal stones), amylase (pancreatitis), glucose (DKA), clotting, group and save/cross-match, lactate and ABG (sepsis management, mesenteric ischaemia).

Imaging includes an erect CXR. Free air under the diaphragm suggests perforated viscus, pneumonia (referred pain) or congestive cardiac failure (CCF; liver congestion). An abdominal X-ray will look for obstruction or IBD.

Urinalysis to look for urinary tract infection (UTI), ketones in DKA, hamaturia in renal stones and a pregnancy test. Perform an ECG (referred pain MI).

Further tests may be guided by the clinical findings and results of investigations thus far, but commonly include USS or CT scan of the abdomen.

Red flag conditions

Ruptured abdominal aortic aneurysm

This is a surgical emergency with a high mortality and should be considered in any patient with a known aneurysm, hypertension or presenting with sudden onset of abdominal pain radiating to the back. The combination of a shocked patient with abdominal pain, or a large drop in haemoglobin in the absence of overt gastrointestinal bleed, should also raise suspicion.

The patient should have two large-bore IV cannulae inserted, bloods sent urgently and cross-matched. O negative blood may be necessary. The surgical team should be contacted immediately. Fluid and blood resuscitation should aim for a systolic BP of 100. There is a role for focussed assessment with sonography for trauma (FAST) scanning in the emergency department, but imaging should not delay surgery.

Ectopic pregnancy

Consider an ectopic pregnancy in all female patients of child-bearing age. Risk factors include previous ectopics, an IUCD, progesterone-only pill and damage to the fallopian tubes (previous endometriosis or salpingitis). Urgent surgery and prompt resuscitation is needed in the case of a ruptured ectopic pregnancy.

Perforated viscus

This arises most commonly from a perforated peptic ulcer, diverticulum or appendix, but gallbladder perforation can occur. It presents with acute abdominal pain, shock, guarding and rebound tenderness with the absence of bowel sounds. Investigations include an erect CXR for the presence of free air under the diaphragm. Keep nil by mouth (NBM), give IV fluids, antibiotics and analgesia. Definitive treatment is prompt surgery.

Appendicitis

Characterized by umbilical pain that localizes to the right iliac fossa. Treatment is appendicectomy followed by IV antibiotics.

TOP TIPS

- Take a thorough history
- Careful examination
- Regular review

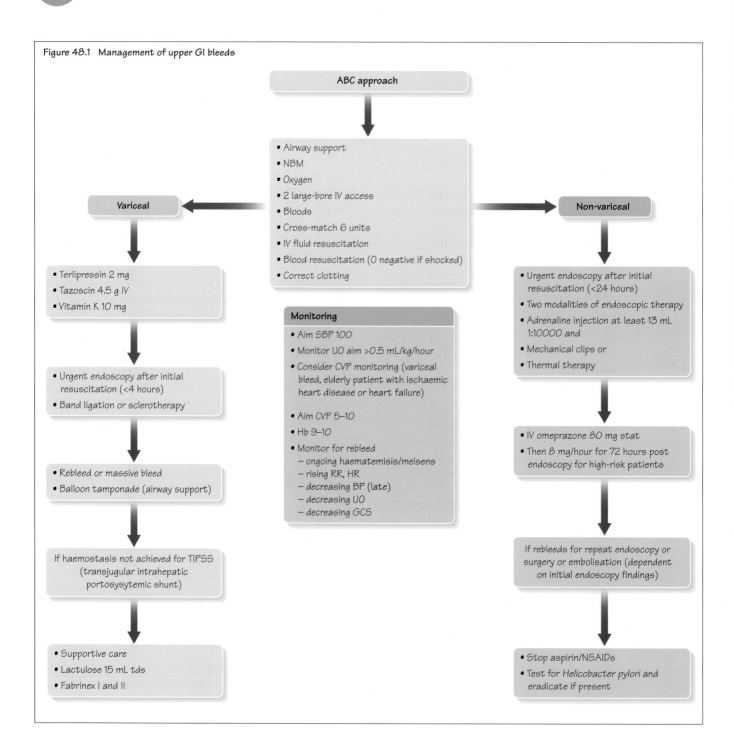

Figure 48.1 Management of upper GI bleeds

ABC approach

- Airway support
- NBM
- Oxygen
- 2 large-bore IV access
- Bloods
- Cross-match 6 units
- IV fluid resuscitation
- Blood resuscitation (0 negative if shocked)
- Correct clotting

Variceal

- Terlipressin 2 mg
- Tazoscin 4.5 g IV
- Vitamin K 10 mg

- Urgent endoscopy after initial resuscitation (<4 hours)
- Band ligation or sclerotherapy

- Rebleed or massive bleed
- Balloon tamponade (airway support)

If haemostasis not achieved for TIPSS (transjugular intrahepatic portosysytemic shunt)

- Supportive care
- Lactulose 15 mL tds
- Fabrinex I and II

Monitoring

- Aim SBP 100
- Monitor UO aim >0.5 mL/kg/hour
- Consider CVP monitoring (variceal bleed, elderly patient with ischaemic heart disease or heart failure)

- Aim CVP 5–10
- Hb 9–10
- Monitor for rebleed
  – ongoing haematemisis/meisens
  – rising RR, HR
  – decreasing BP (late)
  – decreasing UO
  – decreasing GCS

Non-variceal

- Urgent endoscopy after initial resuscitation (<24 hours)
- Two modalities of endoscopic therapy
- Adrenaline injection at least 13 mL 1:10000 and
- Mechanical clips or
- Thermal therapy

- IV omeprazone 80 mg stat
- Then 8 mg/hour for 72 hours post endoscopy for high-risk patients

If rebleeds for repeat endoscopy or surgery or embolisation (dependent on initial endoscopy findings)

- Stop aspirin/NSAIDs
- Test for Helicobacter pylori and eradicate if present

This chapter covers the assessment and management of upper gastrointestinal (GI) tract bleeding.

GI bleeds are divided clinically into upper and lower gastrointestinal bleeding, defined as proximal or distal to the ligament of Trietz. An upper GI bleed is a medical emergency. It can present as haematemesis, melaena, coffee ground vomit, collapse or a shocked patient with a rapid drop in haemoglobin. The presence of fresh PR bleeding with haemo-

dynamic compromise needs to be treated as a fast transit upper GI bleed initially. Overall mortality from an upper GI bleed remains at 10%. Factors associated with a poor prognosis include age, co-morbidities, liver disease, bleed whilst an inpatient (as generally unwell), the presence of shock, haematemesis (as opposed to melaena alone), fresh PR bleeding, ongoing bleeding and raised urea.

Causes

A cause may not be identified in up to 20% of endoscopies in patients presenting with an upper GI bleed but the main causes are shown in Table 48.1.

Table 48.1 The main causes of an upper GI bleed

Cause	Percentage
Peptic ulcer	44%
Oesophagitis	28%
Gastritis/erosions	26%
Erosive duodenitis	26%
Varices	13%
Portal hypertensive gastropathy	7%
Malignancy	5%
Mallory–Weiss tear	5%
Vascular malformations	3%

History

- Have you vomited any blood? Have you passed any blood or black stools?
- Assessing the volumes passed: how many episodes of vomiting? How much did you vomit? Was it fresh blood from the start or did this come later? Was it fresh or altered blood? Were there any blood clots? What colour are your stools? How many times have you passed black stools?
- Assessing shock: have you felt dizzy or light-headed? Any blackouts? Have you felt clammy or short of breath?
- Symptoms that point to a cause: have you had any acid reflux or heartburn (gastritis, oesophagitis)? Any epigastric pain (peptic ulcer disease)? Have you had any difficulty swallowing or weight loss (malignancy)?
- Previous medical history (co-morbidities): to risk stratify. Any chronic liver disease (varices)? Previous peptic ulcer disease? Any previous episodes? Any operations? Any history of AAA or AAA repair (aortoenteric fistula)?
- Medications: ask specifically about aspirin, NSAIDs, warfarin, clopidogrel. Selective serotonin re-uptake inhibitors (SSRIs), bisphosophonates and steroids can increase bleeding risk.

- Social history: alcohol intake? Do you smoke?
- Family history: hereditary haemorrhagic telangiectasia, GI malignancy, liver disease?

Initial assessment and management: the ABC approach

Get senior help early.

(A) Is the airway at risk from vomiting?

(B) Respiratory rate (early sign of shock). Measure oxygen saturations. Listen to the chest – any signs of aspiration? Apply oxygen. Perform an ABG.

(C) Measure HR, BP (including postural BP if lying BP is satisfactory) to assess degree of shock. Check capillary refill time. Insert two large-bore IV access. Take blood for FBC, U&E (disproportionate urea rise due to protein load), LFTs, CRP, amylase, clotting and group and save, and cross-match 4–6 units if the patient is high risk. Commence fluid resuscitation, followed by blood. Use O-negative blood if shocked.

(D) GCS and BM (liver disease).

(E) Check for signs of anaemia and jaundice and for the presence of a liver flap indicating hepatic encephalopathy. Look for evidence HHT, and for signs of weight loss. Abdominal examination may be normal. Check for splenomegaly and ascites (portal hypertension); is there an abdominal mass (malignancy). Perform a PR examination. Catheterize to monitor urine output.

Order an erect CXR and liaise with haematology if blood is anticoagulated or if abnormal clotting to normalize INR. Options may include vitamin K, fresh frozen plasma or beriplex to reverse warfarin. Platelets or cryoprecipitae may also be necessary.

Liaise with a gastroenterologist early regarding timing of endoscopy. Specific management of variceal and non-variceal bleeds is outlined Fig. 48.1.

Calculate the Rockall score to predict mortality (Table 48.2). Postendoscopy score < 3 indicates good prognosis, > 8 poor prognosis.

> **TOP TIPS**
> - Resuscitation
> - Transfusion and correcting clotting
> - Endoscopy for definitive treatment

Table 48.2 The Rockall score

Variable	Score			
	0	1	2	3
Age (years)	< 60	60–79	> 80	
Shock	'No shock' SBP > 100 HR < 100	'Tachycardia' SBP > 100 HR > 100	'Hypotension' SBP < 100	
Co-morbidity	None		CCF, IHD, any major co-morbidity	Renal failure, liver failure, malignancy
Diagnosis	Mallory–Weiss tear, no SRH	All other diagnoses	Malignancy	
Major stigmata of recent haemorrhage	None, or dark spot only		Blood in upper GI tract, adherant clot, visible or spurting vessel	

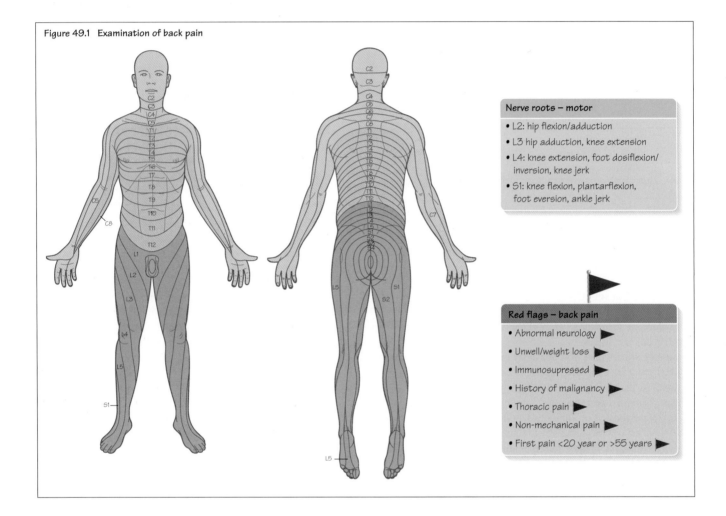

Figure 49.1 Examination of back pain

Nerve roots – motor

- L2: hip flexion/adduction
- L3 hip adduction, knee extension
- L4: knee extension, foot dosiflexion/inversion, knee jerk
- S1: knee flexion, plantarflexion, foot eversion, ankle jerk

Red flags – back pain

- Abnormal neurology
- Unwell/weight loss
- Immunosupressed
- History of malignancy
- Thoracic pain
- Non-mechanical pain
- First pain <20 year or >55 years

This chapter covers the differential diagnosis, investigations and basic treatment of acute back pain and large joint pain.

Back pain

The vast majority of back pain is self-limiting and is dealt with in primary care. Acute back pain can result from a variety of causes.

Differential diagnosis

Trauma

This should be easily identifiable from the history. Musculoskeletal back pain is suggested by pain related to movement and localized tenderness. In the absence of red flag symptoms (Fig. 49.1), over-investigation should be avoided.

Vertebral fracture

Fractures can be related to trauma, malignancy, infection or osteoporosis. A thorough history should help elucidate the underlying cause (e.g. weight loss, fever, osteoporosis risk factors). Suspected fracture is the only indication for performing a plain X-pay.

Neurological symptoms

The majority of cases with a radiculopathy will be related to acute/subacute disc prolapse or foraminal stenosis. Try to determine the nerve root affected (Fig. 49.1). A full neurological examination is required. Straight leg raise above 60° may precipitate pain. Enquire about symptoms suggestive of central cord compression. Cord compression can also be related to malignancy (primary or secondary), infection (discitis) and inflammation. **Remember cord compression is a medical emergency! If suspected an urgent MRI is required.**

Inflammatory back pain

This will rarely present acutely, but may occur acutely in patients with a known inflammatory condition (e.g. reactive spondyloarthropathy, ankylosing spondylitis). Inflammatory back disease usually presents in young patients (15–30 years) and is typically eased with exercise. It may also have associated alternating buttock pain. Whilst plain X-ray can show established deformities, magnetic resonance imaging (MRI) is better in early disease and for detecting active inflammation.

Remember to exclude alternative causes of back pain such as pyelonephritis or aortic aneurysms.

Investigations

• In acute back pain, suspected fracture is the only indication for performing a plain X-ray. Osteoporosis cannot be diagnosed on X-ray, a duel-energy X-ray absorptiometry (DEXA) scan is required
• MRI is the imaging modality of choice in patients with acute back pain with or without red flag symptoms (Fig. 49.1) and for chronic back pain
• CT can be useful for cases in which MRI is contraindicated, and is useful in guiding soft tissue and bone biopsies
• An isotope bone scan is helpful in identifying widespread metastatic bone disease

Treatment

Simple musculoskeletal back pain should be treated with reassurance, physiotherapy and simple analgesia. Excessive bed rest should be avoided. Muscle relaxants such as low-dose diazepam can be a useful adjunct. Specific causes of back pain such as infection, cord compression and malignancy require senior input and referral to the appropriate medical or surgical specialties.

Large joint pain

Acute pain can be divided into poly- and monoarticular presentations. A detailed history should help in differentiating between potential diagnoses.

Polyarthritis

• Flare of inflammatory polyarthritis (IPA)
• Polyarticular crystal arthropathy
• Reactive arthritis

Monoarthritis

• Trauma
• Haemarthrosis
• Septic arthritis
• Crystal arthropathy (urate or calcium pyrophosphate dihydrate disease (CPPD))
• IPA
• Avascular necrosis (AVN)

The hot swollen joint

The differential includes:
• Septic arthritis
• Crystal arthritides
• Reactive arthritis
• Flare of a pre-existing IPA

It is important not to miss a septic joint due to the morbidity and mortality associated with it. Patients are typically unwell with associated fever and an acutely painful swollen joint. Crystal arthropathies are recurrent and self-limiting. A reactive arthritis occurs in the context of recent infection, typically gastrointestinal or genitourinary in origin.

Trauma

Usually identifiable from the history. A haemarthrosis is confirmed on aspirating blood from a swollen painful joint.

Avascular necrosis

Commonly occurs in hip and knee joints. Patients usually have associated risk factors such as prolonged steroid use, alcohol use or previous trauma.

Remember that the structures around joints such as bursa, tendons and cartilage can also be affected, and may be the cause of the 'joint pain'.

Investigations

Routine blood tests including CRP, ESR and serum urate are useful baseline investigations. Blood cultures should be performed in all patients with suspected septic arthritis. If an effusion is present, the joint needs to be aspirated (prosthetic joints should be referred to orthopaedics). Synovial fluid should be sent for Gram stain, culture and sensitivity and crystal microscopy. Remember that urate/CPPD crystals can coexist with sepsis.

Plain X-rays in the acute setting are advised to investigate bony trauma and to assess for chondrocalcinosis (associated with crystal arthropathies). MRI and musculoskeletal ultrasound are helpful in identifying effusions and damage to surrounding tissues. MRI is also the imaging modality of choice for assessing the presence of osteomyelitis.

Treatment

Specific treatment depends on the underlying cause. Rest of the affected joint and analgesia is helpful in most cases. NSAIDs are helpful in the treatment of IPA and crystal arthropathies. If contraindicated, colchicine or steroids (intra-articular, intramuscular or low-dose oral) can be used as alternatives (in the absence of infection). Suspected septic arthritis should be treated as per the local antibiotic protocol until initial culture results are known. If infection is confirmed, antibiotics should be continued for 6 weeks. If patients are not improving despite appropriate antibiotic therapy, referral to orthopaedics for arthroscopic wash-out should be considered. Orthopaedics should also be consulted regarding trauma and AVN.

TOP TIPS

• The majority of acute back pain is self-limiting and does not require detailed investigation
• Always assess for symptoms/signs of cord compression
• Blood cultures should be performed in all patients with suspected septic arthritis
• Whilst joint aspiration prior to antibiotics administration in septic arthritis is preferable, don't delay treatment!

References

BSR & BHPR, BOA, RCGP and BSAC (2006) *Guidelines for the Management of the Hot Swollen Joint in Adults*.
Cush, J.J., Kavanaugh, A.F. & Stein, C.M. (2004) *Rheumatology. Diagnosis and therapeutics*, 2nd edn. Lippincott Williams and Wilkins, Philadelphia.
Hakim, A., Clunie, G. & Haq, I. (2011) *Oxford Handbook of Rheumatology*, 3rd edn. Oxford University Press, Oxford.
National Institute for Health and Care Excellence (NICE) (2009) *Low Back Pain* NICE, London.
Royal College of Radiologists (2012) *Making the Best Use of Clinical Radiology Services*. www.rcr.ac.uk/content.aspx?pageID=995. (last accessed 11 September 2013).

Figure 50.1 Fractures and dislocations

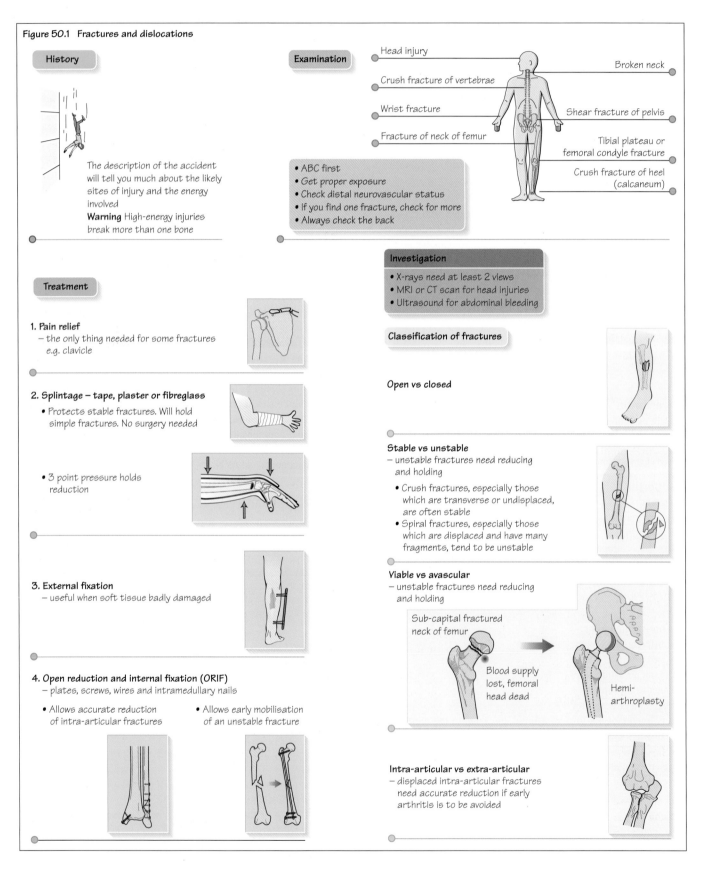

History

The description of the accident will tell you much about the likely sites of injury and the energy involved
Warning High-energy injuries break more than one bone

Examination

Head injury

Crush fracture of vertebrae

Wrist fracture

Fracture of neck of femur

Broken neck

Shear fracture of pelvis

Tibial plateau or femoral condyle fracture

Crush fracture of heel (calcaneum)

• ABC first
• Get proper exposure
• Check distal neurovascular status
• If you find one fracture, check for more
• Always check the back

Investigation

• X-rays need at least 2 views
• MRI or CT scan for head injuries
• Ultrasound for abdominal bleeding

Classification of fractures

Open vs closed

Stable vs unstable
– unstable fractures need reducing and holding

• Crush fractures, especially those which are transverse or undisplaced, are often stable
• Spiral fractures, especially those which are displaced and have many fragments, tend to be unstable

Viable vs avascular
– unstable fractures need reducing and holding

Sub-capital fractured neck of femur

Blood supply lost, femoral head dead

Hemi-arthroplasty

Intra-articular vs extra-articular
– displaced intra-articular fractures need accurate reduction if early arthritis is to be avoided

Treatment

1. Pain relief
   – the only thing needed for some fractures e.g. clavicle

2. Splintage – tape, plaster or fibreglass
   • Protects stable fractures. Will hold simple fractures. No surgery needed

   • 3 point pressure holds reduction

3. External fixation
   – useful when soft tissue badly damaged

4. Open reduction and internal fixation (ORIF)
   – plates, screws, wires and intramedullary nails

   • Allows accurate reduction of intra-articular fractures
   • Allows early mobilisation of an unstable fracture

This chapter covers the assessment and management of injuries (Fig. 50.1).

Causes

If the load on a limb exceeds the strength of the bone, joint capsule or ligaments, then a fracture, dislocation or joint sprain will occur. If the load is normal but the bone is weak, then this is a pathological fracture, e.g. fractured neck of the femur in an elderly female. Repetitive loading may cause a stress fracture as in long-distance runners.

Shape and direction of injury

1 **Shape of the fracture.** This is determined by the direction of force applied:
- Spiral fractures result from twisting
- Crush fractures result from excess longitudinal load
- Transverse fractures result from bending forces
- Very high impact energies tend to explode the bone

2 **Dislocation.** A joint is more susceptible to dislocation if the patient has lax ligaments or if there is damage to the capsule from a previous dislocation.

History

The patient will be able to describe what they have felt or heard. Dislocations may relocate spontaneously, so the patient's description of what happened is valuable.

Examination

Do not forget to check distal neurovascular status, then use the 'look, feel, move' system to check for:
- Wounds on the skin
- Bleeding into the soft tissues
- Deformity of bones and joints

Movement needs to be performed carefully, watching the patient's face, testing for ruptures of muscles and ligaments, instability of joints and even crepitus in bones. Don't forget, if there is enough energy for one injury, then there is plenty for more, so check the whole body.

Investigation

At least two X-rays will be needed centred on the site of injury, aligned at right angles to each other.

Classification of fractures

1 **Open versus closed –** any wound in a limb that is fractured means that we must treat the fracture as if it is open rather than closed. Open fractures are contaminated until otherwise proven. If the wound is not cleaned out at once, then infection will set in. Once infection has established itself in the bone, then it is said that it can never be eradicated – it may always break out again. It is better to prevent **osteomyelitis** than try to cure it. Photograph the wound then cover it to prevent further contamination, give prophylactic antibiotics, and arrange for urgent surgery to clean the wound and close it if possible, once the fracture has been fixed.

2 **Viable versus avascular –** if the fracture pattern results in pieces of bone losing their blood supply, they cannot heal. They may then need removing and/or replacing.

3 **Stable versus unstable –** some fractures (especially those involving a simple crush) are stable. In other cases fractures are unstable, especially spiral or comminuted (multifragmentary) fractures.

4 **Intra-articular versus extra-articular – i**f displaced intra-articular fractures are not reduced exactly (less than a 2 mm step in the articular surface) then **early arthritis** in that joint is inevitable.

Growth plate fractures in children

Fractures across the growth plates of children's bones can interfere with the ability of that bone to grow, and need handling with special care. Every effort must be made to prevent the epiphyseal plate from producing a deformity.

Management

A displaced fracture needs 'reducing' and then 'holding'.

1 **Reduction.** Paradoxically, the first move is to increase the deformity in the direction of the original damaging force. This allows the joint or fracture fragments to be separated from each other without damaging the capsule or periosteum, which is intact on the inside of the deformity. The intact periosteum is then used as the hinge and the guide to bring the structures back into their correct relationship.

2 **Fixation.** Once reduced the fracture or dislocation needs to be held to prevent it displacing again:
- Sometimes a simple sling will be adequate
- In other cases bone fragments may need to be held exactly in position with a plate and screws
- Plaster of Paris is cheap and simple to use but does not hold fractures very precisely and is a great inconvenience to the patient while they wait for the fracture to heal. However, this method may be ideal for fractures in children, which heal quickly and remodel as they grow. If the fracture is unstable, moulding the plaster using three-point pressure may reduce the risk of the fracture slipping
- In patients with fractures through metastases, quick and strong fixation with an intramedullary nail will allow them to get home as quickly as possible

Complications

Fractures can unite in a bad position (**mal-union**) or heal slowly or even not at all (**non-union**). Failure to unite can be a result of poor blood supply. In this case the bone ends just wither away. A little movement stimulates bone healing. Too much movement produces exuberant new bone, but a failure to bridge the cleft. Bone grafting and secure fixation of the fracture may be needed to treat delayed union or non-union.

Stiffness and weakness can be a problem after fractures or dislocations. Physiotherapy has a key role in rehabilitation.

Osteotomies

Bones can be broken deliberately to correct deformity or even to lengthen limbs. External fixator frames can then be used to move fragments of bone, providing the speed is not so high that non-union results or too slow so that the osteotomy unites before adequate movement has been achieved.

TOP TIPS

- Check ABC first, then for other injuries
- Check distal neurovascular status
- Open fractures need cleaning out to prevent osteomyelitis
- Fractures into joints need exact reduction
- Fractures into the growth plates of children's bones need special care
- Pathological fractures in the elderly need quick fixation to return their mobility

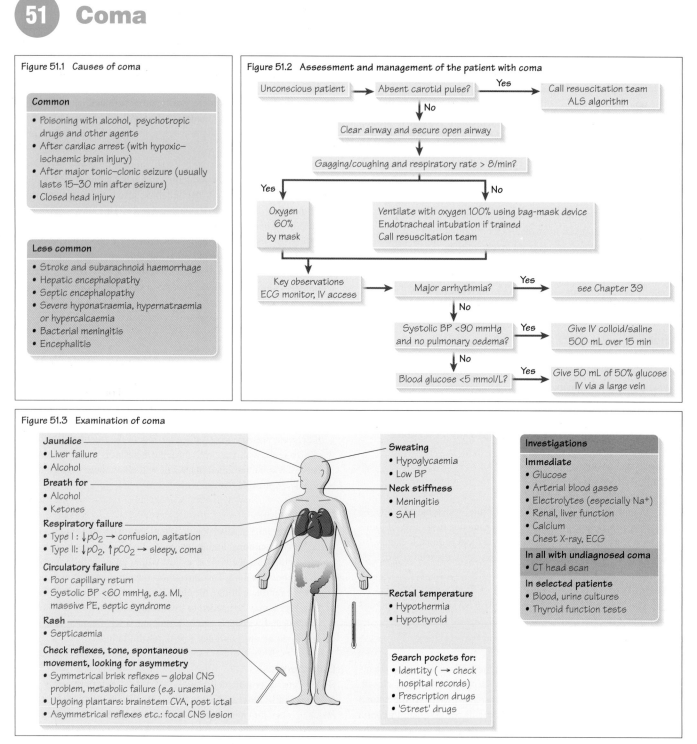

Figure 51.1 Causes of coma

Common

- Poisoning with alcohol, psychotropic drugs and other agents
- After cardiac arrest (with hypoxic–ischaemic brain injury)
- After major tonic–clonic seizure (usually lasts 15–30 min after seizure)
- Closed head injury

Less common

- Stroke and subarachnoid haemorrhage
- Hepatic encephalopathy
- Septic encephalopathy
- Severe hyponatraemia, hypernatraemia or hypercalcaemia
- Bacterial meningitis
- Encephalitis

Figure 51.2 Assessment and management of the patient with coma

Unconscious patient → Absent carotid pulse? → Yes → Call resuscitation team ALS algorithm

↓No

Clear airway and secure open airway

Gagging/coughing and respiratory rate > 8/min?

Yes → Oxygen 60% by mask

No → Ventilate with oxygen 100% using bag-mask device / Endotracheal intubation if trained / Call resuscitation team

Key observations ECG monitor, IV access → Major arrhythmia? → Yes → see Chapter 39

↓No

Systolic BP <90 mmHg and no pulmonary oedema? → Yes → Give IV colloid/saline 500 mL over 15 min

↓No

Blood glucose <5 mmol/L? → Yes → Give 50 mL of 50% glucose IV via a large vein

Figure 51.3 Examination of coma

Jaundice
- Liver failure
- Alcohol

Breath for
- Alcohol
- Ketones

Respiratory failure
- Type I : $\downarrow pO_2 \rightarrow$ confusion, agitation
- Type II: $\downarrow pO_2$, $\uparrow pCO_2 \rightarrow$ sleepy, coma

Circulatory failure
- Poor capillary return
- Systolic BP <60 mmHg, e.g. MI, massive PE, septic syndrome

Rash
- Septicaemia

Check reflexes, tone, spontaneous movement, looking for asymmetry
- Symmetrical brisk reflexes – global CNS problem, metabolic failure (e.g. uraemia)
- Upgoing plantars: brainstem CVA, post ictal
- Asymmetrical reflexes etc.: focal CNS lesion

Sweating
- Hypoglycaemia
- Low BP

Neck stiffness
- Meningitis
- SAH

Rectal temperature
- Hypothermia
- Hypothyroid

Search pockets for:
- Identity (→ check hospital records)
- Prescription drugs
- 'Street' drugs

Investigations

Immediate
- Glucose
- Arterial blood gases
- Electrolytes (especially Na^+)
- Renal, liver function
- Calcium
- Chest X-ray, ECG

In all with undiagnosed coma
- CT head scan

In selected patients
- Blood, urine cultures
- Thyroid function tests

This chapter covers the assessment and immediate management of patients who have lost consciousness. Coma is a medical emergency, because patients in coma are at high risk of permanent brain injury or death, caused either by the underlying disorder or its secondary effects. Immediate action is needed to stabilize the airway, breathing and circulation, and correct hypoglycaemia, while you diagnose and treat the cause.

Causes

The causes of coma you are likely to see are summarized in Fig. 51.1. Coma is usually due to disorders affecting the whole brain, e.g.

poisoning, electrolyte disorders and bacterial meningitis. It may also reflect supratentorial mass lesions with secondary brainstem compression, such as an expanding intracerebral haematoma, and primary disorders of the brainstem. Clinical assessment and neuroimaging with CT will usually allow rapid differentiation between these three groups.

Assessment of the level of consciousness

Consciousness is a continuum from full alertness to complete unresponsiveness. It can be graded clinically using the Glasgow Coma Scale (GCS). Coma is defined as a score of 8 or below, and a reduced conscious level as a score between 9 and 14.

Priorities

- **Stabilize the airway, breathing and circulation**. One of the major risks of impaired consciousness is loss of the ability to protect the airway. As a general rule, patients with a GCS score of 8 or below (P or U on the AVPU scale) should be considered for endotracheal intubation
- **Exclude /treat hypoglycaemia**
- Give **naloxone** if opioid poisoning is possible, and **flumazenil** if the patient has received benzodiazepine in hospital
- **Diagnose and treat the underlying cause**
- **Give supportive care** and prevent the complications of coma (e.g. airway obstruction, pressure necrosis of skin or muscle, corneal abrasions, inhalation pneumonia)

History

Obtain the history from all available sources. Establish:

- The setting and time course of the loss of consciousness. Was loss of consciousness abrupt (e.g. subarachnoid haemorrhage (SAH), seizure), gradual (e.g. poisoning, bacterial meningitis) or fluctuating (e.g. recurring seizures, subdural haematoma, metabolic encephalopathy)?
- If loss of consciousness was preceded by neurological or other symptoms
- The co-morbidities of the patient: systemic (e.g. chronic obstructive pulmonary disease, chronic liver disease), neurological (e.g. major epilepsy) and psychiatric
- A complete list of current medications. If the patient was admitted with coma, find out exactly what medications were being taken prior to admission (contact the patient's GP to check prescribed medications, and ask a family member to collect all medications in the home)
- If there has been previous or recent alcohol or substance abuse
- If there has been recent foreign travel (raising the possibility of infectious diseases acquired abroad, such as falciparum malaria).

Examination

- Document the level of consciousness in objective terms, e.g. GCS
- Assess carefully the respiratory rate and pattern. Hyperventilation may be seen in coma due to ketoacidosis (diabetic or alcoholic); liver failure; renal failure; bacterial meningitis; poisoning with aspirin, carbon monoxide, ethanol, ethylene glycol, methanol, paracetamol or tricyclics; stroke complicated by pneumonia or pulmonary oedema; brainstem stroke
- Examine for signs of head injury (e.g. scalp laceration, bruising, bleeding from an external auditory meatus or the nose). If there are signs of head injury, assume additional cervical spine injury until proven otherwise; the neck must be immobilized in a collar and X-rayed before you check for neck stiffness and the oculocephalic response
- Check for neck stiffness: neck stiffness may be seen in bacterial meningitis, encephalitis, SAH, cerebral or cerebellar haemorrhage with extension into the subarachoid space, and cerebral malaria. However, in any of these conditions, neck stiffness may be lost with increasing depth of coma
- Check the position of the eyes, the size and symmetry of the pupils and their response to bright light. With the exception of coma due to opioid poisoning (characterized by pinpoint pupils), normal pupils indicate a toxic/metabolic cause for coma
- Check the corneal reflex: a normal response bilaterally (eyelid closure and upward deviation of the eyes) indicates normal function of the midbrain and pons. The corneal reflex may be lost in deep coma due to metabolic encephalopathy or poisoning
- Check the oculocephalic response: this is a simple but important test of an intact brainstem. Rotate the head to the left and right. In an unconscious patient with an intact brainstem, both eyes rotate counter to the movement of the head
- Examine the limbs: tone, response to a painful stimulus (nailbed pressure), tendon reflexes and plantar responses
- Examine the fundi: spontaneous venous pulsation excludes raised intracranial pressure. Subhyaloid haemorrhages may be seen in SAH
- Complete a systematic examination of the patient: check for possible complications of coma (e.g. pressure necrosis of the skin or muscle, corneal abrasions, inhalation pneumonia)

Urgent investigation of the unconscious patient

The investigations are set out in Fig. 51.1. The following additional investigations should be undertaken if indicated:

- ECG if there is hypotension, coexistent heart disease or suspected ingestion of cardiotoxic drugs (antiarrhythmics, tricyclics)
- Plasma osmolality if poisoning is suspected or coma remains unexplained. The normal range of plasma osmolality is 280–300 mosmol/kg. If the measured plasma osmolality (by freezing point depression method) exceeds the calculated osmolality (from the formula $[2(Na + K) + urea + glucose]$) by 10 mosmol/kg or more, consider poisoning with ethanol, ethylene glycol, isopropyl alcohol or methanol
- Prothrombin time if liver failure is suspected or coma unexplained
- Blood culture if temperature is < 36 or $> 38°C$
- Blood for toxicology screen (including paracetamol) if poisoning is suspected or cannot be excluded
- Cranial CT if:
  - Coma followed a fall or head injury
  - Focal neurological signs
  - Papilloedema or other evidence of raised intracranial pressure
  - No systemic cause for the coma is apparent
- Lumbar puncture (assuming no contraindication on CT) if:
  - Meningitis or encephalitis are suspected.
  - SAH is suspected, but CT is normal
- Electroencephalograph (EEG) if:
  - Non-convulsive status epilepticus is suspected
  - Encephalitis is suspected
  - No cause for the coma is found

Further management

Patients with coma should be nursed in a high-dependency or intensive care unit. The level of consciousness should be monitored using the GCS, with observations initially every 15–30 minutes. As well as specific treatment directed at the underlying cause, supportive care of the comatose patients includes stabilization of the airway, breathing and circulation, correction of hypoglycaemia or hyperglycaemia, treatment of seizures if present, correction of fever or hypothermia, and prevention of the complications of coma.

TOP TIPS

- Coma is a medical emergency
- Use a systematic approach to identifying and reversing the cause

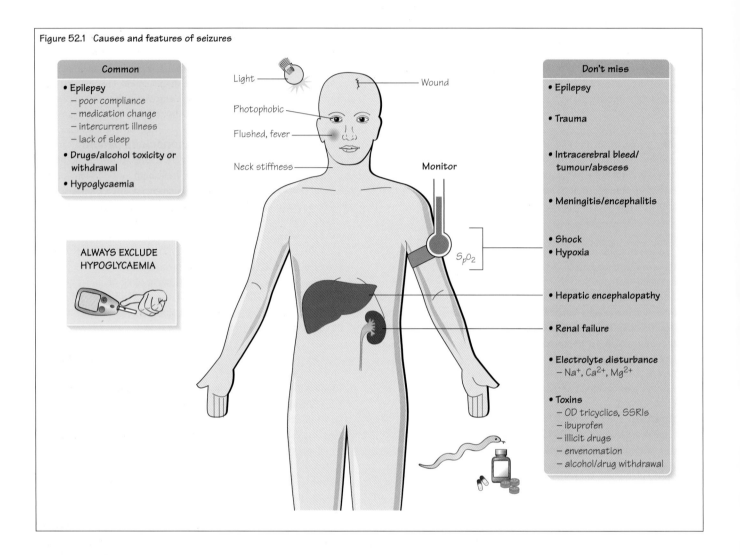

Figure 52.1 Causes and features of seizures

Common
- Epilepsy
  - poor compliance
  - medication change
  - intercurrent illness
  - lack of sleep
- Drugs/alcohol toxicity or withdrawal
- Hypoglycaemia

ALWAYS EXCLUDE HYPOGLYCAEMIA

Light
Photophobic
Flushed, fever
Neck stiffness
Wound
Monitor
S_pO_2

Don't miss
- Epilepsy
- Trauma
- Intracerebral bleed/tumour/abscess
- Meningitis/encephalitis
- Shock
- Hypoxia
- Hepatic encephalopathy
- Renal failure
- Electrolyte disturbance
  - Na^+, Ca^{2+}, Mg^{2+}
- Toxins
  - OD tricyclics, SSRIs
  - ibuprofen
  - illicit drugs
  - envenomation
  - alcohol/drug withdrawal

This chapter covers the investigation and treatment of the convulsing patient. In addition, it provides guidance on what should be communicated to the patient and their carers about the impact on the activities of daily living.

Seizures are the result of electrical 'storms' in the brain. Most seizures occur in people with known epilepsy: these patients often do not come to hospital unless the seizure is different from their normal pattern, or occurs in public. Most seizures last less than 5 minutes, so will have finished by the time the patient reaches A&E.

In a generalized or tonic-clonic seizure, the patient loses consciousness, their body tenses (tonic phase) and then undergoes a series of rhythmic contractions affecting all their muscles (clonic phase). Partial seizures exhibit a wide spectrum of patterns of motor activity and sensory disturbance according to the area of brain affected.

Primary seizures occur in patients with no underlying pathological cause. Secondary seizures occur as a result of some pathophysiological process.

Stop the seizure

The ABC rules apply, but with caveats. Never try to splint or force the mouth open. Patients may be cyanosed during the active phases of seizures, but if there is upper airway obstruction try a nasopharyngeal airway. Key points are:
- Ensure the patient will not hurt themselves while fitting
- Give oxygen 100% by reservoir mask
- Check blood sugar – if below 4 mmol/L, give 50 mL of 50% dextrose IV or 1 mg IM glucagon

First line: benzodiazepines

If intravenous access is available, use the doses as listed under 'Second line' below, otherwise give:
- Midazolam 10 mg buccal **or**
- Diazepam 10 mg rectal

Second line: benzodiazepines

If the first dose of benzodiazepine has not terminated the seizure after 10 minutes, give a further dose of benzodiazepine:

- Lorazepam 4 mg IV **or**
- Diazepam 10 mg IV

If the patient is dependent on alcohol, give high-dose intravenous thiamine to prevent long-term brain damage.

Third line: anticonvulsants

Phenytoin (or the prodrug fosphenytoin) is given as a loading dose over 30 minutes and then (if necessary) as a continuous infusion. Patients already taking phenytoin do not need a loading dose. Phenytoin is a sodium channel blocker with cardiac effects, so ECG and blood pressure must be monitored during use; contraindications include cardiac conduction problems or significant heart failure.

Fourth line: sedation and intubation

A generalized seizure lasting over 30 minutes, or recurrent seizures within 30 minutes without return of consciousness, is described as status epilepticus. If such convulsions continue for more than 60 minutes despite treatment this is 'refractory status epilepticus' and the patient should be sedated and intubated to control the seizure, and transferred to the ITU.

After the seizure: the post-ictal period

After a generalized seizure has finished, it is normal for the patient to be unconscious for a few minutes, longer with high doses of benzodiazepines. When consciousness returns, it is common for the patient to be transiently confused, agitated and sometimes aggressive. Partial seizures may have little or no post-ictal period.

Search for a cause
Was it a seizure?

A good witness history is critical. Other differential diagnoses are:

- Syncope/collapse (see Chapter 65)
- Hypoxia, metabolic causes – hyponatraemia, hypocalcaemia
- Toxic causes

Seizure vs pseudoseizure

Pseudoseizures ('non-epileptic attacks') can be very difficult to differentiate from generalized seizures; about 25% of patients intubated for 'seizures' are having a pseudoseizure. Pseudoseizures are more likely if there are asymmetrical movements, pelvic thrusting, head rolling, resistance to eye opening or no post-ictal period. In pseudoseizures, incontinence is unusual and tongue biting, if it occurs, involves the tip rather than the sides of the tongue that one would expect in a generalized seizure. The reasons for pseudoseizures are usually complex and the labelling has significant risks, so should only be confirmed by a senior doctor.

Causes, triggers and auras

In a person with known epilepsy, common causes are non-compliance, changed dose of anticonvulsant or drug interactions (Fig. 52.1). Alcohol or benzodiazepine withdrawal causes seizures. Triggers are factors that may cause fits in people who are not normally prone to fits (e.g. lack of sleep, infections). An aura is the feeling that a patient with epilepsy has that warns them that a seizure is imminent.

Examination

Look for head trauma, injuries occurring as a result of the seizure, signs of sepsis/systemic illness or toxicity. Any suspicion of a rash or neck stiffness should prompt immediate antibiotics for meningitis.

Cardiovascular examination is particularly important because cardiac causes are common differential diagnoses in the young (tachyarrhythmias, hypertrophic obstructive cardiomyopathy (HOCM)) and the elderly (bradyarrhythmias, postural hypotension, valvular disease). Collapse due to cardiac causes may be accompanied by a few seconds of jerking limbs due to transient inadequate brain perfusion – 'anoxic jerks'.

Neurological examination after the post-ictal period is often normal, but if there are focal neurological signs, this should prompt further investigation, e.g. CT. Immediately after a generalized seizure, the plantar reflexes may be up-going, and there may be ankle clonus. Todd's palsy is a transient unilateral weakness following a seizure that resolves over a few hours, but can be difficult to differentiate from a transient ischaemic attack (TIA)/stroke.

Investigations

- **Bedside investigations**: blood glucose, ECG
- **Laboratory investigations**:
  ○ FBC, U&E, calcium
  ○ Anticonvulsant levels – not always helpful but should be performed if toxicity is suspected (e.g. patient is ataxic)
  ○ Prolactin rises after a seizure – the sample should be taken between 10 and 20 minutes after the seizure, but should only be ordered if the diagnosis is unclear
- **Imaging**: CT is indicated for a first seizure or abnormal neurology

Who can go home?

- **Known epilepsy**: if the seizure is within the patient's normal pattern, they have a full recovery, and will be with a responsible adult, discharge is likely to be safe
- **'First fit'**: patients not previously known to be epileptic should be observed for at least 4 hours. If no serious underlying cause is found and there are no complications, they may be discharged. On discharge they must be advised – and this must be recorded in the notes – to avoid any activity in which a further fit would be dangerous (e.g. driving, operating machinery, climbing ladders, unsupervised swimming) until they have been reviewed by a specialist. Outpatient clinic follow up should be organized following EEG and CT

TOP TIPS

- Protect the convulsing patient from harm and give oxygen
- Refer new patients for specialist follow up
- Record advice about activities of daily living

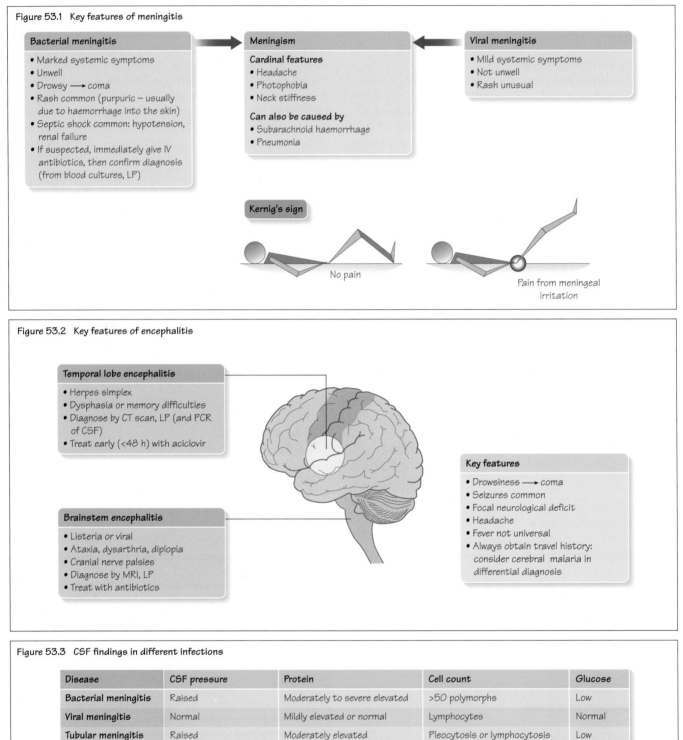

Figure 53.1 Key features of meningitis

Bacterial meningitis
- Marked systemic symptoms
- Unwell
- Drowsy ⟶ coma
- Rash common (purpuric – usually due to haemorrhage into the skin)
- Septic shock common: hypotension, renal failure
- If suspected, immediately give IV antibiotics, then confirm diagnosis (from blood cultures, LP)

Meningism

Cardinal features
- Headache
- Photophobia
- Neck stiffness

Can also be caused by
- Subarachnoid haemorrhage
- Pneumonia

Viral meningitis
- Mild systemic symptoms
- Not unwell
- Rash unusual

Kernig's sign

No pain

Pain from meningeal irritation

Figure 53.2 Key features of encephalitis

Temporal lobe encephalitis
- Herpes simplex
- Dysphasia or memory difficulties
- Diagnose by CT scan, LP (and PCR of CSF)
- Treat early (<48 h) with aciclovir

Brainstem encephalitis
- Listeria or viral
- Ataxia, dysarthria, diplopia
- Cranial nerve palsies
- Diagnose by MRI, LP
- Treat with antibiotics

Key features
- Drowsiness ⟶ coma
- Seizures common
- Focal neurological deficit
- Headache
- Fever not universal
- Always obtain travel history: consider cerebral malaria in differential diagnosis

Figure 53.3 CSF findings in different infections

Disease	CSF pressure	Protein	Cell count	Glucose
Bacterial meningitis	Raised	Moderately to severe elevated	>50 polymorphs	Low
Viral meningitis	Normal	Mildly elevated or normal	Lymphocytes	Normal
Tubular meningitis	Raised	Moderately elevated	Pleocytosis or lymphocytosis	Low
	Normal			
Encephalitis	Raised or normal	Mildly elevated or normal	Lymphocytosis	Normal
Malignant meningitis	Mildly raised or normal	Raised	Raised: either reactive lymphocytes or malignant cells	Low

This chapter covers the common infections affecting the central nervous system (CNS). These include meningitis, encephalitis and cerebral abscess. The immunocompromised, such as those with human immunodeficiency virus (HIV), are at particular risk of these infections.

Meningitis

Acute meningitis presents with fever, headache, stiff neck and photophobia, and can be caused by bacteria or viruses (Fig. 53.1).

Bacterial meningitis

Bacterial meningitis is often associated with a septic syndrome (fever, tachycardia, hypotension or shock, complicated by septicaemia-induced disseminated intravascular coagulation). Meningitis is usually secondary to bacteraemia caused by *Neisseria meningitidis*, although *Streptococcus pneumoniae* occurs in those with pneumococcal pneumonia (more common in elderly people and those who abuse alcohol) or damaged dura (skull fracture, ear sepsis, sinus disease).

Once bacterial meningitis is suspected, broad-spectrum antibiotics (e.g. high-dose ceftriaxone) must be given immediately (i.e. in the community if necessary).

The diagnosis is confirmed by identifying the organism using blood culture, cerebrospinal fluid (CSF) (Fig. 53.1), microscopy, culture and polymerase chain reaction (PCR) or blood serology.

The prognosis is variable. In meningococcal meningitis, 5–10% die, and a significant proportion have permanent sequelae, including loss of digits (infarction secondary to hypotension), deafness, blindness and intellectual impairment. Immunization against meningococcal serotype A and C is effective (but serotype B, against which there is no vaccine, now accounts for 90% of cases in the UK).

Listeria monocytogenes causes meningitis in susceptible individuals (pregnant women, people with alcohol problems, immunocompromised individuals), with a rapidly progressive picture resembling brainstem encephalitis with focal signs and meningism. Treatment is with ampicillin.

Viral meningitis

Viral meningitis presents with prominent headache and less obvious signs of meningeal irritation than in bacterial infections. The responsible organism is identified (CSF, PCR or serology) in only 50% of cases, and is often an enterovirus.

Many of the common childhood viral infections, including measles and chickenpox, may be accompanied by a meningitic illness which, although usually mild, can rarely be life threatening.

Management is symptomatic with rehydration and analgesia.

Other causes of meningitis

• **Non-infective causes of meningism** (i.e. headache, photophobia and stiff neck) include subarachnoid haemorrhage and migraine (although this requires exclusion of more serious diagnoses)
• **Malignant meningitis** usually presents with sequential cranial nerve palsies, initially painless and later painful, but can cause meningism. Spinal nerve root involvement also occurs
• **Meningoencephalitis** is meningitis plus some parenchymal involvement

• **Tubercular meningitis or cryptococcal meningitis**: a chronic presentation may occur and these are more common in the immunocompromised. Tubercular meningitis is increasing in frequency in the West

Encephalitis

Encephalitis implies infection of the brain substance itself. This is rare. The clinical picture is of fever, headache and a diffuse (i.e. confusion, drowsiness up to coma) rather than focal disturbance of cerebral function. The onset may be very dramatic over just a few hours, although more usually the history extends back several days. Other features include seizures, wandering, behavioural change and frank psychiatric syndromes.

The diagnosis is made from the combination of suggestive clinical features and a lymphocytosis in the CSF. Supportive data come from finding focal inflammation on CT/MRI, focal slow wave activity on EEG and detection of the organism (culture, PCR, serology). There are a large number of viruses responsible, with a marked geographical variation (e.g. Japanese B in the Far East, western equine in the USA) so a travel history is vital. A cause is only identified in 30% of cases. The prognosis is variable.

The principal treatable cause is herpes simplex encephalitis, which accounts for 20% of viral encephalitis and has the following features:
• Presents with a viral prodrome followed by behavioural changes with amnesia and sometimes dysphasia
• Rapid evolution to coma may occur
• EEG shows repetitive epileptic discharges localized to the temporal lobes
• CT/MRI shows necrotizing inflammation in the temporal lobes
• Treatment is with immediate high-dose aciclovir
• Prognosis is poor and long-term sequelae are common: 10% die acutely, 10% are so severely impaired as to be rendered institutionalized, 20% are left dependent, and 60% recover but in the majority formal neuropsychological testing reveals residual deficits and most do not function at their pre-morbid occupational level

Cerebral abscess

Cerebral abscess is rare and presents with headache, fever and focal neurological signs. Infection arises from direct spread (e.g. infected ears, sinuses) or from infected emboli (endocarditis, cyanotic congenital heart disease).

First-line investigation is with CT/MRI. Lumbar puncture (LP) must not be performed because the risk of 'coning' (i.e. herniation of the brain through the foramen magnum, precipitating coma and death) is high. Organisms are cultured from the blood or pus aspirated from the abscess. Echocardiography to exclude cardiac infection should be undertaken.

Treatment is with prolonged antibiotics and sometimes neurosurgical drainage. The mortality rate is 25%.

TOP TIPS

• Maintain a high index of suspicion for meningitis
• Wherever possible take a full history including recent travel

Figure 54.1 Main features of stroke and transient ischaemic attack

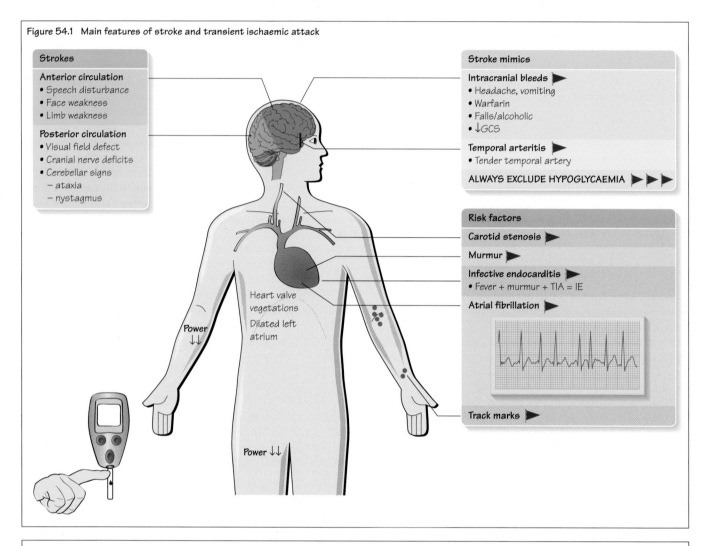

Strokes

Anterior circulation
- Speech disturbance
- Face weakness
- Limb weakness

Posterior circulation
- Visual field defect
- Cranial nerve deficits
- Cerebellar signs
  - ataxia
  - nystagmus

Stroke mimics

Intracranial bleeds ▶
- Headache, vomiting
- Warfarin
- Falls/alcoholic
- ↓GCS

Temporal arteritis ▶
- Tender temporal artery

ALWAYS EXCLUDE HYPOGLYCAEMIA ▶ ▶ ▶

Risk factors

Carotid stenosis ▶

Murmur ▶

Infective endocarditis ▶
- Fever + murmur + TIA = IE

Atrial fibrillation ▶

Track marks ▶

Heart valve vegetations

Dilated left atrium

Power ↓↓

Power ↓↓

Figure 54.2 ABCD2 score for TIA

Clinical detail	Score
Age >60 years	1
Blood pressure >140/90	1
Clinical features:	
Unilateral weakness	2
Speech disturbance without weakness	1
Duration:	
>60 mins	2
10–60 mins	1
Diabetes	1
Total >4 = high risk – need urgent investigation	
Total >5 = 8% risk of stroke in next 48 hours	

This chapter covers the assessment and management of patients with cerebrovascular accidents (stroke). Stroke is a major cause of mortality and chronic disability. The advent of thrombolysis for stroke has prompted campaigns to increase public awareness of stroke symptoms, e.g. 'FAST – face, arm, speech, time to call ambulance'. Stroke thrombolysis in carefully selected patients reduces disability in survivors. Strokes can be prevented by identification, investigation and treatment of TIA patients at high risk of stroke.

Clinical assessment

The time of onset, type and duration of symptoms is critical to decision making. Many patients have an indistinct onset of stroke symptoms (e.g. have woken with symptoms) and are therefore ineligible for thrombolysis. History and examination should cover:

- Time of onset
- Risk factors for atherosclerosis (diabetes, smoking, hypertension, ↑cholesterol, family history)
- Risk factors for embolism, e.g. atrial fibrillation (AF), valvular disease, coagulopathy (Fig. 54.1)
- Contraindications to thrombolysis
- A brief but thorough neurological examination
- Consider stroke mimics

Investigations

1 **Bedside investigations:**
   - Blood glucose
   - ECG
2 **Laboratory investigations:**
   - FBC, U&E, clotting
3 **Imaging:**
   - Immediate CT/MRI to exclude haemorrhage if inside thrombolysis window. Unconscious patients may need intubation to perform CT safely
   - Chest X-ray

Stroke

A stroke is defined as a 'focal neurological deficit of cerebrovascular cause that persists beyond 24 hours'.

Stroke subtypes: clinical syndromes

- *Anterior circulation infarction* (40%): limb weakness combined with visual field loss and/or cortical dysfunction (e.g. aphasia/apraxia) suggests a partial (20%) or complete (20%) cortical infarction. If the dominant hemisphere is affected, aphasia and apraxia are common, whereas involvement of the non-dominant hemisphere gives contralateral hemi-neglect
- *Lacunar infarction* (30%) of the internal capsule results in motor/sensory loss affecting two or more of the face, arm and leg *without* visual or speech disturbance
- *Posterior circulation infarction* (15%): visual problems and/or cerebellar symptoms (ataxia, nausea/vomiting) and cranial nerve deficits are the hallmark of a posterior infarction, although weakness and sensory deficits may also occur
- *Haemorrhage* (15%): intracerebral (10%) and subarachnoid (5%). Warfarin therapy, early vomiting, severe headache, drowsiness and hypertension are common in these patients

Stroke mimics

- *Hypoglycaemia* must be excluded on arrival. Hypoglycaemia can give a strikingly similar clinical picture to stroke, is easy to diagnose and treat, and if untreated will result in significant neurological damage
- *Seizures* may give a transient hemiplegia – 'Todd's palsy'
- Recent trauma or falls suggest *subdural* haematoma
- Fever suggests *infection*, e.g. sepsis, meningitis, encephalitis, brain abscess, septic emboli
- A history of cancer warrants exclusion of brain *metastases* using CT with contrast
- *Migraine* can give a transient hemiparesis, visual, speech or sensory symptoms
- *Giant cell arteritis*: suspect if there is visual disturbance in patients over 50 years old. Check for tender temporal artery and raised ESR
- Isolated lower motor neuron facial weakness could be due to *Bell's palsy*. Symmetrical normal forehead movement ('raise your eyebrows') implies an upper rather than a lower motor neuron deficit. Inflammation affecting the facial nerve gives unilateral facial muscle weakness. Although most cases will resolve over a few weeks, prednisolone for 10 days improves recovery if started within 3 days of onset. Inability to close the eye needs ophthalmology review
- *Functional* (psychological/psychiatric) disorders may present as stroke, e.g. somatization

Treatment

Ischaemic stroke

Patients with ischaemic stroke, confirmed by clinical symptoms and absence of bleeding on CT, *and* who are less than 3 hours from symptom onset are eligible for thrombolysis. After establishing absence of contraindications and obtaining informed consent, thrombolysis is performed with tissue plasminogen activator (tPA).

If the patient has an ischaemic stroke but is not eligible for thrombolysis, aspirin should be started immediately. To prevent aspiration, patients should have a swallowing assessment before being given food or drink. Pressure area care and adequate hydration are essential in immobile patients.

Haemorrhagic stroke

Intracranial bleeding in patients on anticoagulants has a poor prognosis, and must be rapidly halted using fresh frozen plasma or prothrombin complex concentrate (expensive) and vitamin K. Surgical treatment should be considered.

Transient ischaemic attack

A TIA is a focal CNS disturbance caused by transient brain ischaemia from emboli or thrombosis with *complete resolution* within 24 hours. This can make differentiation from stroke difficult; patients with a neurological deficit that is resolving spontaneously should not receive thrombolysis.

The ABCD^2 score estimates the short-term risk of stroke (Fig. 54.2). Patients with high scores must be investigated and treated urgently to prevent a stroke, e.g.:
- Carotid stenosis – endarterectomy
- Atrial fibrillation, cardiac failure – anticoagulation

Antiplatelet therapy (e.g. aspirin) should be started immediately if a TIA is suspected and there are no contraindications.

TOP TIPS

- Exclude hypoglycaemia
- Urgently investigate patients with TIAs who have high ABCD scores

---

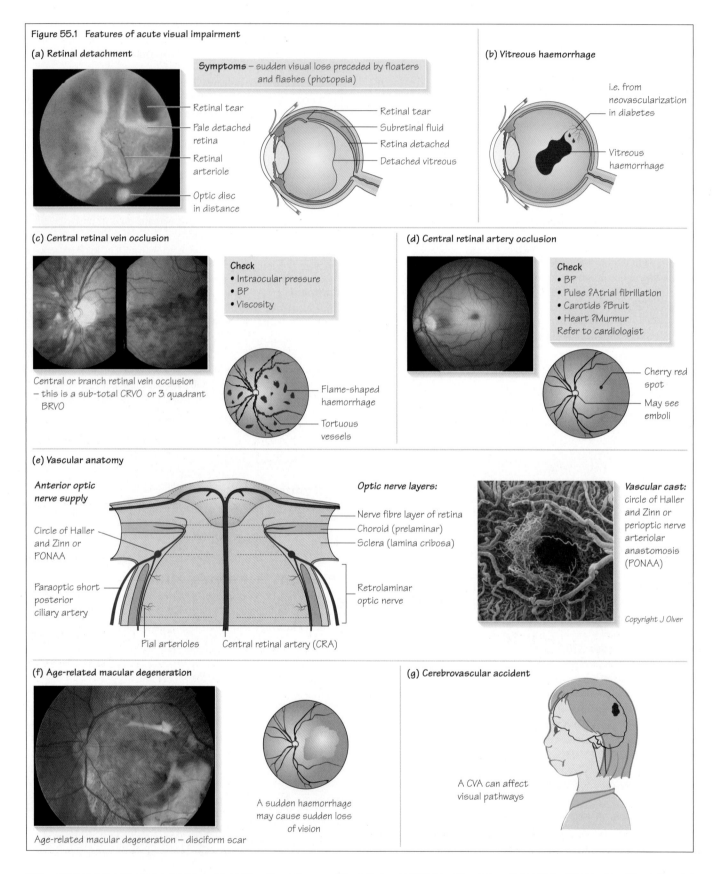

Figure 55.1 Features of acute visual impairment

(a) Retinal detachment

Symptoms – sudden visual loss preceded by floaters and flashes (photopsia)

- Retinal tear
- Pale detached retina
- Retinal arteriole
- Optic disc in distance

- Retinal tear
- Subretinal fluid
- Retina detached
- Detached vitreous

(b) Vitreous haemorrhage

i.e. from neovascularization in diabetes

Vitreous haemorrhage

(c) Central retinal vein occlusion

Check
- Intraocular pressure
- BP
- Viscosity

Central or branch retinal vein occlusion – this is a sub-total CRVO or 3 quadrant BRVO

- Flame-shaped haemorrhage
- Tortuous vessels

(d) Central retinal artery occlusion

Check
- BP
- Pulse ?Atrial fibrillation
- Carotids ?Bruit
- Heart ?Murmur
Refer to cardiologist

- Cherry red spot
- May see emboli

(e) Vascular anatomy

Anterior optic nerve supply

Circle of Haller and Zinn or PONAA

Paraoptic short posterior ciliary artery

Pial arterioles   Central retinal artery (CRA)

Optic nerve layers:
- Nerve fibre layer of retina
- Choroid (prelaminar)
- Sclera (lamina cribosa)
- Retrolaminar optic nerve

Vascular cast: circle of Haller and Zinn or periopic nerve arteriolar anastomosis (PONAA)

Copyright J Olver

(f) Age-related macular degeneration

Age-related macular degeneration – disciform scar

A sudden haemorrhage may cause sudden loss of vision

(g) Cerebrovascular accident

A CVA can affect visual pathways

This chapter covers the main causes of painless acute visual impairment. These are: vascular occlusion of the retina, optic nerve or brain; acephalgic migraine; vitreous haemorrhage; and retinal detachment (Fig. 55.1).

Vascular occlusion

Retinal vein occlusion

Central retinal vein occlusion (CRVO) or branch retinal vein occlusion (BRVO) presents with sudden unilateral painless loss of vision. The diagnosis is made on ophthalmoscopic appearance, which shows multiple blot and flame retinal haemorrhages. It is caused by: systemic hypertension, hyperviscosity, vessel wall disease such as diabetes or inflammation (e.g. sarcoidosis) or raised intraocular pressure.

Assessment and management

• As CRVO and BRVO are strongly associated with arteriosclerosis, BP must be checked and evidence of arterial disease elsewhere sought (determine from the history whether there are any symptoms of myocardial infarction, stroke or claudication; feel all the pulses, listen for arterial bruits)
• Check intraocular pressure
• Check for diabetes and systemic inflammation
Younger patients presenting with CRVO or BRVO, especially those with a past history or family history of thrombosis, or older patients in whom there is no obvious cause, should be investigated for hyperviscosity syndromes or thrombophilia.

Retinal artery occlusion

Central retinal artery occlusion or branch retinal artery occlusion also present as acute, painless, unilateral loss of vision. The ophthalmoscope shows pale retinal ischaemia, perhaps with a foveal cherry-red spot, and may show a retinal embolus.

Causes include: arterial embolus from diseased carotid, left-sided valvular heart disease, left ventricular mural thrombus, or AF with a left atrial thrombus.

Assessment and management

• Examine the patient carefully, considering that some part of the 'arterial organ' is damaged
• Control risk factors and if appropriate consider carotid endarterectomy, aspirin or cardiac intervention

Non-arteritic anterior or posterior ischaemic optic neuropathy

This form of occlusion is usually painless, unlike the arteritic form associated with giant cell arteritis, which is usually associated with headache or jaw pain. Visual loss may be altitudinal – loss of top or bottom half of visual field – often in stepwise episodes.
• In anterior ischaemic optic neuropathy (AION) the optic disc is swollen. Swelling may be segmental or involve the entire nerve head. There are often associated splinter haemorrhages on the disc
• In posterior ischaemic optic neuropathy (PION) the optic disc looks normal
It is caused by occlusion of the small ciliary vessels supplying the optic nerve head (AION) or posterior optic nerve (PION). Risk factors include smoking, arteriosclerosis, hypertension, a hypotensive episode or a 'disc at risk' – a small optic nerve head with no central cup.

Assessment and management

• Arteritis must be ruled out with normal erythrocyte sedimentation rate and C-reactive protein. Consider a referral for a temporal artery biopsy if in doubt
  ◦ Control risk factors
  ◦ Unlike the arteritic form, corticosteroids have no place in the management

Cerebrovascular accident

A haemorrhagic or embolic CVA affecting the posterior visual pathways – radiation or cortex – will present as acute, painless visual loss. Depending on the site of the lesion, the patient will have a corresponding contralateral, homonymous hemi or quadrantic field defect to confrontation. It is rare for the visual loss to be the only symptom.

Acephalgic migraine

This form of migraine presents with transient visual disturbance involving both eyes, in the absence of headache. A blind spot or flickering light evolves over about 20 minutes, and then subsides.

Vitreous haemorrhage

Haemorrhage into the vitreous cavity can result in sudden painless loss of vision. The extent of visual loss will depend on the degree of haemorrhage:
• A large haemorrhage may cause almost total unilateral visual loss
• A small haemorrhage presents as floaters with normal, or only slightly reduced, visual acuity
  Causes include:
• Proliferative retinopathy with spontaneous rupture of abnormal fragile new vessels that grow on the retinal surface; the most common cause is diabetes
• Warfarin may predispose
• Vitreous or retinal detachment – a small retinal blood vessel may rupture when the retinal break occurs
• Trauma
• Posterior vitreous detachment can result in vitreous haemorrhage if, as the vitreous separates from the retina, it pulls and ruptures a small blood vessel

Management

Refer to an ophthalmologist to determine cause and manage accordingly.

Retinal detachment

• Sudden, or rapid, painless loss of vision
• Often preceded by symptoms of flashing lights (photopsia) and/or floaters and/or visual field defect
• When the macula is not involved, the visual loss involves the peripheral field and visual acuity may be normal
• Once the macula is involved, the central vision is lost

Management

Refer to an ophthalmologist to consider laser to a retinal tear or retinal surgery ± vitrectomy (surgery to remove some or all of the vitreous humour) for a full detachment.

TOP TIPS

• Take a full history and consider risk factors
• Remember to look in the eyes with an ophthalmoscope

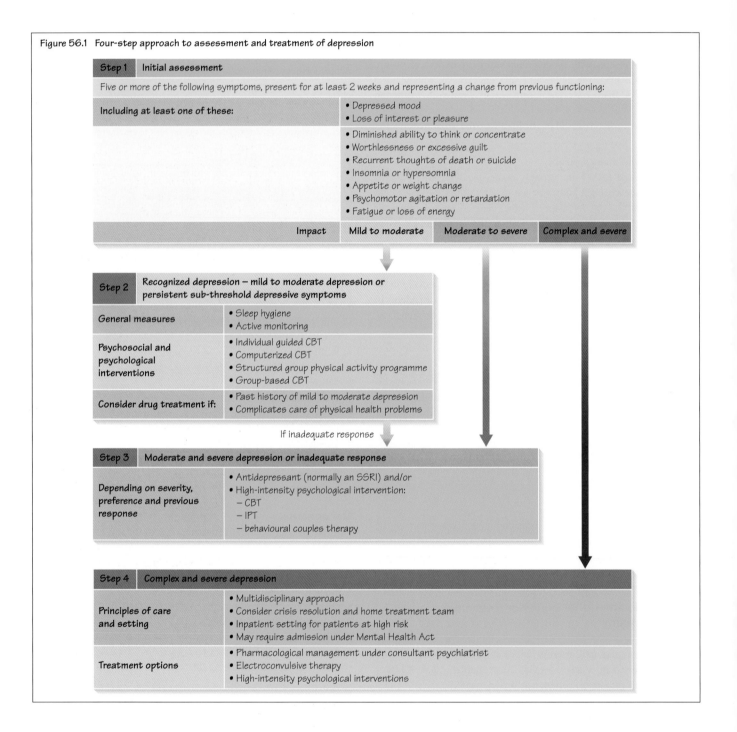

Figure 56.1 Four-step approach to assessment and treatment of depression

Step 1 Initial assessment

Five or more of the following symptoms, present for at least 2 weeks and representing a change from previous functioning:

Including at least one of these:	• Depressed mood • Loss of interest or pleasure
	• Diminished ability to think or concentrate • Worthlessness or excessive guilt • Recurrent thoughts of death or suicide • Insomnia or hypersomnia • Appetite or weight change • Psychomotor agitation or retardation • Fatigue or loss of energy

Impact	Mild to moderate	Moderate to severe	Complex and severe

Step 2 Recognized depression – mild to moderate depression or persistent sub-threshold depressive symptoms

General measures	• Sleep hygiene • Active monitoring
Psychosocial and psychological interventions	• Individual guided CBT • Computerized CBT • Structured group physical activity programme • Group-based CBT
Consider drug treatment if:	• Past history of mild to moderate depression • Complicates care of physical health problems

If inadequate response

Step 3 Moderate and severe depression or inadequate response

Depending on severity, preference and previous response	• Antidepressant (normally an SSRI) and/or
	• High-intensity psychological intervention:
	  – CBT
	  – IPT
	  – behavioural couples therapy

Step 4 Complex and severe depression

Principles of care and setting	• Multidisciplinary approach • Consider crisis resolution and home treatment team • Inpatient setting for patients at high risk • May require admission under Mental Health Act
Treatment options	• Pharmacological management under consultant psychiatrist • Electroconvulsive therapy • High-intensity psychological interventions

This chapter covers the diagnosis and management of patients with major depressive episodes. It briefly addresses the aetiology and prognosis of depression and the assessment of risk including the risk of self-harm.

Depression is the second leading cause of disability in the developed world. Approximately one in 40 people meet the diagnostic criteria for a major depressive episode at any one time and almost one in five people will experience an episode at some stage in their lives; 15% of patients with severe depression commit suicide and the risk of suicide following a suicide attempt is 100 times higher compared to the general population. It is essential that all doctors retain a high index of suspicion for this treatable illness.

How to diagnose a major depressive episode

There are three factors to take into account when considering whether or not someone has depression:

1 Type and number of symptoms – depression is a disorder of mood, although it is possible for a depressed patient only to experience loss of enjoyment or interest. At least one of the two core features is required for a diagnosis of a major depressive episode and at least four other features shown in Fig. 56.1.

2 Duration of symptoms – these characteristic symptoms represent a change in normal experience and must be present most of the time for at least 2 weeks. It may be appropriate to make a diagnosis of a depressive episode after a shorter period of time if the patient is experiencing psychotic symptoms (delusions, hallucinations).

3 Impact on day to day activities – patients with mild depressive episodes will experience some impairment at work, socially or in some other important area of their functioning. At the other end of the spectrum, patients with severe episodes of depression may be bed-bound or unable to eat and drink.

What are the risk factors for depression?

You should consider the following predisposing factors for depression as part of your assessment:

- **Female** – affects women:men in a ratio of 2:1
- **Family history**
- **Chronic physical illness**
- **Past history of depression**
- **Lack of a confiding relationship**

  Severe physical illness and loss events (e.g. loss of a job or relationship) can also precipitate a depressive episode.

What are the risks associated with depression?

- **Self-harm/suicide** – you must ask all patients who you are assessing for depression whether they have:
  - Feelings of hopelessness
  - Thoughts of wanting to harm themselves
  - Made any plans to harm themselves, e.g. hoarded pills, bought rope, written a note
- **Harm to others** – although homicide is rare in the context of depression you should ask about thoughts of wanting to harm others. In particular ask about thought of harm to children in women who develop severe depressive symptoms following childbirth
- **Deterioration in physical and mental state**
- **Abuse** (especially in the elderly)

What else could it be?

Major depressive episodes can be confused with other conditions. You should consider the following before making a diagnosis of a major depressive episode:

- **Secondary depression** (e.g. hypothyroidism, Cushing's syndrome, Addison's disease, hyperparathyroidism, alcohol dependence) – the symptoms will only improve if this underlying condition is treated
- **Bipolar depression** – if the patient has had a previous episode of elevated mood (i.e. hypomania or mania) you should discuss treatment options with a psychiatrist as this history is suggestive of bipolar disorder
- **Schizophrenia and schizoaffective disorder** – severe depression with psychotic features should be distinguished from schizoaffective disorder and schizophrenia
- **Adjustment disorder** – mild depressive symptoms should be distinguished from an adjustment disorder or bereavement where onset of symptoms is within 3 months of the life event

How to manage patients with a depressive episode

The management plan depends on the severity of the symptoms and the associated risks. NICE recommends a stepped care approach to the management of depression (Fig. 56.1)

The recognition of patients with major depressive episodes is key (step 1). The majority of patients with depression will be managed in primary care and the exact treatment will depend on the patient's preferences (steps 2 and 3). Patients with severe depressive episodes with or without psychotic features, those at elevated risk of self-harm or suicide, and those with moderately severe depression that has failed to respond to treatment will require the services of a community mental health team, crisis team or admission (step 4). Irrespective of the treatment setting, it is essential that the patient's GP is involved in the care plan.

The treatment options include:

1 Low- or high-intensity psychological interventions:
- Cognitive behavioural therapy (CBT) – a structured treatment that aims to change dysfunctional beliefs, negative automatic thoughts and behaviour. It can be delivered by computer, individually or in a group setting
- Interpersonal therapy (IPT) – a standardized form of brief psychotherapy that looks at the person's interpersonal functioning and identifies the problems associated with the onset of the depression. A trained therapist is required

2 Biological interventions:
- Pharmacotherapy – the choice of antidepressant will depend on the patient's preferences, co-morbid physical health problems and previous response. A SSRI is typically used as the first-line agent. Patients at risk of suicide and those under the age of 30 should be reviewed weekly initially
- Electroconvulsive therapy (ECT) – this is only used for patients with severe depression and will typically require admission

What is the prognosis?

- Untreated episodes typically last between 3 and 8 months
- 20% of patients remain depressed for 2 years or more
- About 50% of patients experience a recurrence
- Recurrent episodes tend to become more severe with shortening disease-free intervals

---

TOP TIPS

- Maintain a high index of suspicion
- Always assess the patient's suicide risk
- Consider other possible conditions
- Involve the patient's GP in the treatment plan, especially when planning discharge

Figure 57.1 Initial assessment and management of psychosis and schizophrenia

First psychotic episode

- Refer urgently to mental health team (e.g. early intervention service, crisis team, community mental health team)
  - consider how to keep the patient safe until initial assessment
  - treatment with antipsychotic medication should only be initiated if directed by mental health team (or GP)
  - physical examination should be conducted prior to commencing treatment

Relapse of schizophrenia

- Refer to mental health team
  - crisis teams can support people with schizophrenia during an acute episode in the community

Promoting recovery

- Monitor physical health (typically in primary care)
  - particular attention to cardiovascular risk
  - ensure results are shared between GP and mental health team
- Re-refer to mental health team if:
  - poor treatment response
  - non-adherence
  - unacceptable side effects
  - risk to the patient or other

This chapter covers the initial assessment and management of patients with psychotic symptoms and in particular schizophrenia. It will be especially relevant to foundation doctors working in the general hospital or primary care.

Managing and reducing the risk of harm to others is also considered. However, it should be remembered that patients with mental health problems, including psychosis, are far more likely to harm themselves than to harm others.

What is psychosis?

Psychosis describes symptoms and signs that reflect a break down in the person's connectedness with reality, e.g.:

- Hallucinations in any sensory modality
- Delusions
- Disorganized speech
- Grossly disorganized behaviour

Psychotic symptoms occur in a range of illnesses including delirium, drug intoxication or withdrawal, mood disorders and schizophrenia.

Schizophrenia

Schizophrenia is a psychotic disorder that presents in a range of different ways. Approximately 1 in 200 people suffer from schizophrenia. In addition to the more florid symptoms (positive symptoms like hallucinations and delusions), patients with schizophrenia often experience loss of normal functioning (or negative symptoms). These negative symptoms include:

- Flattening of mood
- Social withdrawal
- Lack of motivation
- Loss of pleasure

For a diagnosis of schizophrenia, the characteristic symptoms should be present most of the time for 1 month.

How to assess for psychosis

When assessing someone with a suspected psychotic episode in the general hospital or in primary care, you should first consider your own safety. This may mean that you make the assessment with someone else present, that you have a safety alarm and that you can easily exit the assessment room. You should discuss how to approach such an assessment with your supervisor.

There are three important sources of information:

- The patient's notes (if available) or referral – this may help guide how you undertake the assessment
- The patient's history and mental state examination
- Information from a relative, family member, carer or other informant (e.g. ambulance crew, police)

Your initial assessment should include an assessment of risk both to the patient (from self-harm, neglect or abuse) and to others. If you need to refer the patient to a specialist mental health service, you should consider how to keep the patient safe until the patient can be reassessed.

Differential diagnosis for schizophrenia

The most common differential diagnoses for a patient presenting with a psychotic episode include:

- Acute intoxication with drugs
- Withdrawal from drugs (including alcohol)
- Delirium

How to manage a patient with schizophrenia

Figure 57.1 describes the recommended approach depending on the phase of the patient's illness – first episode, relapse and promoting recovery.

Treatments include antipsychotic medication and psychological or psychosocial interventions. Antipsychotic medication will typically be initiated by a psychiatrist and may be administered as oral medication or injection (depot). It is vital that the patient's physical health needs are also considered. This means that a thorough physical examination should be conducted prior to initiating treatment. Investigations should include an ECG if specified by the antipsychotic drug product characteristics, if the patient has high blood pressure, if there is a past history of cardiovascular disease or if the patient is being admitted as an inpatient.

The physical health of patients with schizophrenia should be reviewed at least once a year with a particular focus on cardiovascular disease risk (e.g. lipids, diabetes).

Prognosis and risk

Following a first episode of psychosis, 20% of patients recover, 70% have a relapsing disease and 10% are seriously disabled by the disease.

Patients with schizophrenia have a high risk of suicide – the 20-year suicide rate is between 14% and 22%. Patients with schizophrenia are much more likely to harm themselves than others. However, up to 10% of violent crime is perpetrated by people suffering from schizophrenia.

Assessing and managing aggressive patients

Violence in healthcare settings is typically (although not always) related to a physical or psychiatric condition. The best predictor of future violence is past violence. Other risk factors include male sex, history of substance misuse and a current psychotic illness.

Remember, coming into hospital can be very stressful. Every attempt should be made to identify vulnerable patients, acknowledge their stress and create a caring atmosphere responsive to their individual needs.

Recognizing aggression

You should be vigilant to the early warning signs. Initial signs could include agitation or even a change in facial expression. The next level includes threats and curses, followed by physical aggression towards objects, surroundings and, ultimately, other people.

History from others

When faced with an aggressive or violent patient, you should gather as much background information as possible. This should include a verbal report from the nursing staff, the patient's relative and the notes. In particular, you should ascertain:

- Reason for admission to hospital
- Medical history
- Timeline since admission, including any medical or surgical procedures
- Any past psychiatric history, including psychotropic medications
- Alcohol or drug abuse
- Timing of the onset of aggression, whether this was gradual or sudden and any obvious precipitants, e.g. medication

Assessment of the patient

Your safety is paramount. Observation from a distance can provide clues about the general mental state of the patient and the level of confusion, e.g. unsteady gait and a lack of sense of direction, targeted aggression or generalized verbal aggression and violence. It may be necessary to call the police or hospital security before attempting any further assessment.

If safe to do so, you could approach the patient. After introducing yourself, you should make a rapid assessment of the patient's mental state, level of consciousness and the patient's own understanding of the situation.

Management

You should consult a senior colleague when thinking about the management of a situation involving aggression. This could include the psychiatrist on call. Management strategies include trying to calm the patient, providing reassurance and redirecting them to a calmer space. If the level of risk is high and other strategies have failed, it may be necessary to consider sedation. You should follow your hospital's protocol or guideline when considering the use of medication to sedate the patient.

Follow-up

Once the immediate risk has been dealt you should carry out a more thorough assessment to establish a possible cause. Ongoing monitoring of the patient is essential.

TOP TIPS

- Keep yourself safe
- Always consider the patient's needs and preferences
- Seek help from the mental health team
- Remember the patient's physical health needs

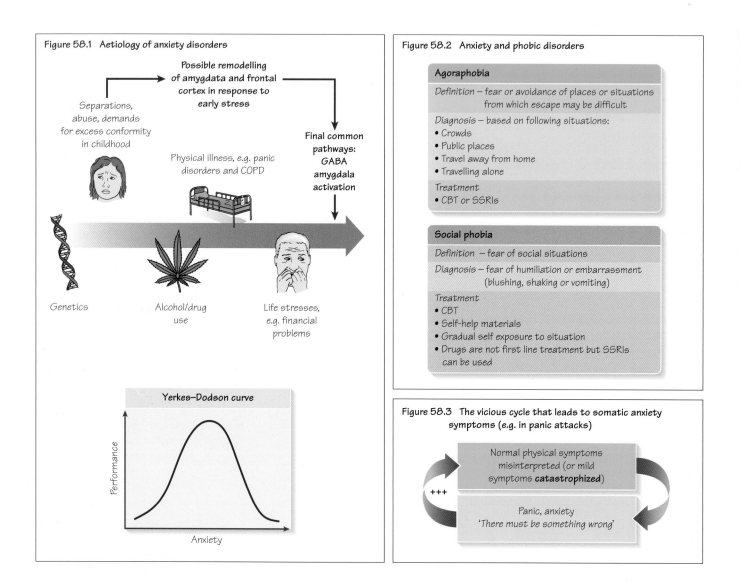

Figure 58.1 Aetiology of anxiety disorders

Possible remodelling of amygdata and frontal cortex in response to early stress

Separations, abuse, demands for excess conformity in childhood

Physical illness, e.g. panic disorders and COPD

Final common pathways: GABA amygdala activation

Genetics

Alcohol/drug use

Life stresses, e.g. financial problems

Yerkes–Dodson curve

Performance

Anxiety

Figure 58.2 Anxiety and phobic disorders

Agoraphobia

Definition – fear or avoidance of places or situations from which escape may be difficult

Diagnosis – based on following situations:
• Crowds
• Public places
• Travel away from home
• Travelling alone

Treatment
• CBT or SSRIs

Social phobia

Definition – fear of social situations

Diagnosis – fear of humiliation or embarrassment (blushing, shaking or vomiting)

Treatment
• CBT
• Self-help materials
• Gradual self exposure to situation
• Drugs are not first line treatment but SSRIs can be used

Figure 58.3 The vicious cycle that leads to somatic anxiety symptoms (e.g. in panic attacks)

Normal physical symptoms misinterpreted (or mild symptoms **catastrophized**)

+++

Panic, anxiety 'There must be something wrong'

It is important to have an understanding of anxiety and phobic disorders as they may mask or mimic physical illnesses and have a huge impact on the patient's life and lifestyle. This chapter covers the common causes of the disorders and their management.

Anxiety is an unpleasant emotional state involving subjective fear, bodily discomfort and physical symptoms. There is often a feeling of impending threat or death, which may or may not be in response to a recognizable threat.

The Yerkes–Dodson curve shows that anxiety can be beneficial up to a plateau of optimal function, beyond which, with increasing anxiety, performance deteriorates.

Anxiety disorders

Pathological anxiety can involve:
• Generalized anxiety, as in generalized anxiety disorder (GAD)

• Discrete anxiety attacks caused by an external stimulus (in phobias) or without external stimulus (in panic disorder)

Anxiety disorders may present alone, but are also frequently co-morbid with other disorders including depression, substance misuse or another anxiety disorder. Anxiety also occurs in other disorders such as depression.

Epidemiology

• Around 6% of the general population have an anxiety disorder at one time. The anxiety disorders comprise:
  • GAD (2–4%)
  • Panic disorder (1%)
  • Phobias (agoraphobia, social phobia, specific phobias)
  • Obsessive–compulsive disorder
• Anxiety disorders are more common in women, younger adults and the middle-aged

- Lower rates are reported in young men and older people; in older people this may be due to the difficulty in detecting anxiety with standard measures

Aetiology (Fig. 58.1)

Biological
- Low levels of γ-aminobutyric acid GABA, a neurotransmitter that reduces activity in the CNS, contribute to anxiety
- Mouse studies have found that the frontal cortex and amygdala undergo structural remodelling induced by the stress of maternal separation and isolation, which alters behavioural and physiological responses in adulthood
- Heightened amygdala activation occurs in response to disorder-relevant stimuli in post-traumatic stress disorder, social phobia and specific phobia
- The medial prefrontal cortex, insula and hippocampus have also been implicated
- Alcohol and benzodiazepine abuse can worsen or cause anxiety and panic attacks

Genetics
- First-degree relatives of people with an anxiety disorder have a quadrupled risk of developing an anxiety disorder
- Some of this risk is disorder-specific and some is not:
  - The genetic factors of panic attacks appear to overlap with depression by about 50%
  - GAD and depression are genetically related
- For social phobia and agoraphobia, genetic risk appears to be mainly due to inheritance of personality traits (low extraversion and high neuroticism)
- Inheritance of specific phobias appears to be independent of personality

Childhood
There is an association with childhood abuse, separations, demands for high achievement and excessive conformity.

Stress
- Anxiety disorder can arise in response to life stresses such as financial problems or chronic disease
- Anxiety disorders are precipitated and perpetuated by physical health problems:
  - A degree of anxiety when facing physical illness, especially when the diagnosis is unclear, is normal
  - Concerns about incontinence, or being ill when out, may perpetuate agoraphobia
  - Panic disorder is ten times more common in people with chronic obstructive airways disease, probably because breathlessness precipitates the symptoms of panic

Panic disorder
- There are current, episodic, severe panic (anxiety) attacks, which occur unpredictably and are not restricted to any particular situation
- Both classificatory systems (DSM-IV-TR and ICD-10) stipulate that at least three panic attacks in a 3-week period should occur for a diagnosis of panic disorder to be made
- Panic attacks are discrete periods of intense fear, impending doom or discomfort, accompanied by characteristic symptoms:
  - Palpitations, tachycardia
  - Sweating, trembling, breathlessness
  - Feeling of choking
  - Chest pain/discomfort
  - Nausea/abdominal discomfort
  - Dizziness, paraesthesia
  - Chills, hot flushes
  - Derealization, depersonalization
  - Fear of losing control, 'going crazy' or dying
- Typically, the episodes only last a few minutes. 'Anticipatory fear' of having a panic attack may develop, with consequent reluctance to be alone away from home
- According to the cognitive model, panic attacks occur when catastrophic misinterpretations of ambiguous physical sensations (e.g. shortness of breath, increased heart rate) increase arousal, creating a positive feedback loop that results in panic
- Selective serotonin re-uptake inhibitors (SSRIs) and cognitive behavioural therapy (CBT) or self-help materials based on CBT principles are recommended first-line treatments
- Tricyclic antidepressants (imipramine, clomipramine) may be helpful where SSRIs are ineffective
- Benzodiazepines are not recommended

Generalized anxiety disorder (GAD)
- GAD is characterized by generalized, persistent, excessive anxiety or worry (apprehensive expectation) about a number of events (e.g. work, school performance) that the individual finds difficult to control, lasting for at least 3 weeks (according to ICD-10) or 6 months or longer (according to DSM-IV-TR). The anxiety is usually associated with:
  - Subjective apprehension (fears, worries)
  - Increased vigilance
  - Feeling restless and on edge
  - Sleeping difficulties (initial/middle insomnia, fatigue on waking)
  - Motor tension (tremor, hyperactive deep reflexes)
  - Autonomic hyperactivity (e.g. tachycardia)
- GAD may be co-morbid with other anxiety disorders, depression, alcohol and drug abuse
- Differential diagnoses include:
  - Withdrawal from drugs or alcohol
  - Excessive caffeine consumption
  - Depression
  - Psychotic disorders
  - Organic causes such as thyrotoxicosis, parathyroid disease, hypoglycaemia, phaeochromocytoma and carcinoid syndrome
- CBT and SSRIs are the recommended first-line treatments
- CBT (self-help material or face to face) for GAD seeks to:
  - Identify morbid anticipatory thoughts and replace them with more realistic cognitions
  - Distraction, breathing and relaxation exercises
- Benzodiazepines should not usually be used beyond 2–4 weeks. Other pharmacological treatments include:
  - Serotonin noradrenaline re-uptake inhibitors (SNRIs)
  - Buspirone
  - Pregabalin

TOP TIPS
- Patients may present with physical symptoms
- Remember there may be co-morbidities
- Patient may be reluctant to explore the issue
- Check for family history of condition
- Ask what help they have already received
- Exclude physical illness

Figure 59.1 The alcohol use disorders identification test: interview version

- Read questions as written. Record answers carefully
- Begin the AUDIT by saying 'Now I am going to ask you some questions about your use of alcoholic beverages during this past year'
- Explain what is meant by 'alcoholic beverages' by using local examples of beer, wine, vodka, etc.
- Code answers in terms of 'standard drinks'. Place the correct answer number in the box at the right

1. How often do you have a drink containing alcohol?

(0) Never [skip to Qs 9 and 10]
(1) Monthly or less
(2) 2 to 4 times a month
(3) 2 to 3 times a week
(4) 4 or more times a week

2. How many drinks containing alcohol do you have on a typical day when you are drinking?

(0) 1 or 2 *
(1) 3 or 4
(2) 5 or 6
(3) 7, 8 or 9
(4) 10 or more

3. How often do you have six or more drinks on one occasion?

(0) Never *
(1) Less than monthly
(2) Monthly
(3) Weekly
(4) Daily or almost daily

4. How often during the last year have you found that you were not able to stop drinking once you had started?

(0) Never
(1) Less than monthly
(2) Monthly
(3) Weekly
(4) Daily or almost daily

5. How often during the last year have you failed to do what was normally expected from you because of drinking?

(0) Never
(1) Less than monthly
(2) Monthly
(3) Weekly
(4) Daily or almost daily

6. How often during the last year have you needed a first drink in the morning to get yourself going after a heavy drinking session?

(0) Never
(1) Less than monthly
(2) Monthly
(3) Weekly
(4) Daily or almost daily

7. How often during the last year have you had a feeling of guilt or remorse after drinking?

(0) Never
(1) Less than monthly
(2) Monthly
(3) Weekly
(4) Daily or almost daily

8. How often during the last year have you been unable to remember what happened the night before because you had been drinking?

(0) Never
(1) Less than monthly
(2) Monthly
(3) Weekly
(4) Daily or almost daily

9. Have you or someone else been injured as a result of your drinking?

(0) No
(2) Yes, but not in the last year
(4) Yes, during the last year

10. Has a relative or friend or a doctor or another health worker been concerned about your drinking or suggested you cut down?

(0) No
(2) Yes, but not in the last year
(4) Yes, during the last year

* Skip to Questions 9 and 10 if total score for Questions 2 and 3 = 0

Record total of specific items here

Around one in four people use alcohol in a harmful way. This means that their pattern of drinking directly leads to physical or mental health problems. Alcohol can cause cancer of the mouth, oesophagus and larynx. Long-term and high use can lead to cirrhosis of the liver and pancreatitis. It aggravates common medical conditions such as hypertension and gastritis and increases the severity of depression.

One in 25 people aged between 16 and 65 are dependent on alcohol. Dependence on alcohol is characterized by a preoccupation with alcohol, craving and a need to drink more to experience the same effect (tolerance). People who are alcohol dependent continue to drink despite experiencing physical, mental or social complications.

This chapter covers the assessment and management of people with harmful drinking or alcohol dependence in community and hospital settings.

Screening for harmful use/alcohol dependence

You should use a validated questionnaire such as the WHO Alcohol Use Disorder Identification Test (AUDIT) when assessing the nature and severity of alcohol misuse (Fig. 59.1). AUDIT was developed to screen for excessive drinking. It will help you identify people who would benefit from reducing or stopping drinking.

There are recommended actions if your patient scores 8 or more:

Score	Recommended action
≥8	Suggestive of harmful alcohol use – consider referral for psychological intervention, e.g. cognitive behavioural therapy, behavioural therapy, couples therapy
>15	Undertake a more detailed assessment
≥20	Detailed assessment and assess for assisted alcohol withdrawal (also consider assisted alcohol withdrawal if patient drinks more than 15 units per day)

Detailed assessment

There are two priorities when assessing a patient with an alcohol use disorder:

1 Severity of associated health and social problems including risk to self and others.

2 Need/appropriateness for assisted alcohol withdrawal.

Your assessment should cover the following:

- Alcohol use, including consumption (historical and recent patterns of drinking)
- History of epilepsy
- Withdrawal-related seizures or delirium tremens
- Other drug misuse, including over-the-counter medication
- Physical health problems especially cardiovascular disease or chronic liver disease
- Psychological problems including depression or psychosis
- Social problems
- Cognitive function (e.g. mini mental state examination)
- Readiness and belief in ability to change

Blood tests may be necessary to help identify or assess for the severity of physical health problems, e.g. liver function tests.

Depending on the extent of the alcohol use and severity of the dependence on alcohol, you should refer to a specialist alcohol service for assisted withdrawal. If the patient is already an inpatient, you should follow your hospital guideline for managing alcohol withdrawal. The key principles of assisted alcohol withdrawal are described below.

Management of assisted alcohol withdrawal

If you are working in general practice or in outpatients, you should consider referring patients who typically drink over 15 units of alcohol per day and/or who score 20 or more on AUDIT to a specialist alcohol services. The decision to manage the withdrawal in the community or in an inpatient setting will be determined by the severity of dependence and co-morbid physical or psychiatric illnesses.

Vulnerable patients (e.g. cognitive impairment, older adults, homeless) and patients who have a history of epilepsy or withdrawal-related seizures or delirium tremens will typically require inpatient treatment.

Alcohol withdrawal in hospital

Alcohol withdrawal is characterized by at least two of the following:

- Autonomic hyperactivity (e.g. sweating or pulse rate greater than 100 bpm)
- Increased hand tremor
- Insomnia
- Nausea or vomiting
- Transient visual, tactile or auditory hallucinations or illusions
- Psychomotor agitation
- Anxiety
- Grand mal seizures

The symptoms start within hours of stopping or reducing drinking. Delirium develops 2–3 days later and usually lasts 48–72 hours. You should also watch for the effects of other illnesses and infection as well as withdrawal from other drugs.

Patients will often complain of withdrawal symptoms but have no objective evidence of withdrawal. Objective assessment is essential.

Constant assessment and support from nursing staff is vital to safely manage patients who are withdrawing from alcohol. This is particularly important to reduce the risk of the patient suffering injury when confused. Confusion tends to be worst at night. Patients should be cared for in well-lit rooms.

You should follow local guidelines for the management of patients withdrawing from alcohol. These may use either a fixed dose or symptom triggered regimen. Benzodiazepines are the mainstay of treatment and these are generally reduced over 7–10 days.

You should also give parenteral thiamine followed by oral thiamine if the patient is malnourished, at risk of malnourishment or has liver disease.

TOP TIPS

- Use a structured tool to assess for alcohol misuse, e.g. AUDIT
- Be vigilant for the symptoms and signs of alcohol withdrawal
- Follow your hospital's guideline for managing alcohol withdrawal

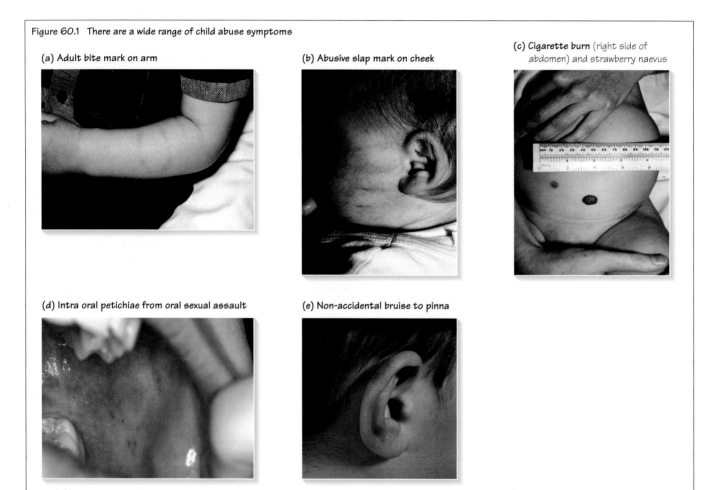

Figure 60.1 There are a wide range of child abuse symptoms

(a) Adult bite mark on arm

(b) Abusive slap mark on cheek

(c) **Cigarette burn** (right side of abdomen) and strawberry naevus

(d) Intra oral petichiae from oral sexual assault

(e) Non-accidental bruise to pinna

Child abuse remains a very topical and controversial subject. This chapter covers the presentation, pitfalls and referral agencies when dealing with a suspected case.

Children in need of safeguarding may present in a wide range of ways (Fig. 60.1), including bruising, fractures, abdominal injury, genital injuries, subdural haemorrhage, immersion type scalds (being dunked in a hot bath), deliberate burns (e.g. cigarette, hot spoon), faltering growth, inadequate supervision or healthcare (e.g. lacking immunizations, severe dental caries), developmental delay, challenging or sexualized behaviour, alleging abuse, pregnant or with sexually transmitted disease following sexual abuse.

The doctor should assess whether a child may be at risk of neglect or abuse as an intrinsic part of every child's assessment, and should also be aware that parental mental health problems may contribute.

Cause for concern – the child's injury

- Presents late or as an incidental finding (e.g. unsuspected fracture)
- Injury does not seem consistent with the explanation given
- No explanation offered by parents or carers
- Explanation changes
- Explanation is not corroborated by others
- Explanation seems incompatible with the child's developmental stage (especially bruising in a non-mobile child)
- Specific patterns of injury (e.g. cigarette burn, glove and stocking scalds suggesting dunking, slap marks, adult bites, genital injury, patterned bruising suggesting use of an implement)

Parental responsibility

Ask who has parental responsibility for the child (and thus the capacity to give consent). Unmarried fathers named on the birth certificate since 1 December 2003 automatically have parental responsibility; a parent's partner may not have. Ask routinely about household composition and relationships.

History

- Check the family history, including any family members with easy bruising or bleeding, or any significant inheritable disorders

- Take a full medical history, including birth history or complications, any bleeding from the cord, neonatal vitamin K, neonatal period, early feeding and development, child health surveillance and immunizations, medication and allergies, hospital admissions and attendances, any other health professionals giving care, and school attendance
- Ask specifically whether the child (or any siblings) is (or was) on the child protection register, and in what category (physical, sexual, emotional, neglect). Ask about any domestic violence (children can be injured physically if 'caught in the crossfire', but also experience emotional abuse by seeing or hearing such violence)
- Ask about general well being, (behaviour, eating, sleeping, toileting, school attendance), recent illness, high temperature, diarrhoea, urinary symptoms, vomiting or rash, any epileptic convulsions, constipation, abdominal pain, abnormal bleeding or bruising

Examination

- Do a full systemic examination
- Look at every part of the body, especially the face and eyes (fundi if possible), earlobes and mastoid areas, inside the mouth, frenum of upper lip, neck, shoulders, chest, back, buttocks, limbs, fingers and toes and external genitalia (with child's consent if age appropriate)
- Note the site, surface appearance and measurements of any bruises, marks or skin lesions including petichiae. Confirm that all bruises/petichiae are non-blanching. Note down the specific explanation for each mark, including when the parent first noticed it

Distinguishing accidental from non-accidental injuries

- Children often have accidents and get bruises, sprains and fractures
- Accidental bruises are usually on bony prominences, especially the forehead and bridge of nose (a blow here can cause bilateral black eyes), chin, shins and knees
- Accidents are typically promptly presented, and explained with a consistent and detailed story, so you get a clear 'video' narrative of how the injury happened and the child's reaction
- Non-accidental injuries tend to have no clear account of causation, the details of how, when, where, who else was present, etc. being sketchy and unclear, with little account of the child's distress or reaction
- This may because the parent or carer is withholding details, or because they were not present when the injury happened (which might implicate them in neglect or another adult in causing an injury)

Action

- Take a careful history and do a full examination, including face, buttocks, fingers and toes
- Write down the account given for the injury, and its aftermath, noting who (including the child) gave the account and when
- If you are unsure, discuss your concerns with your senior before discharge
- If necessary, take advice from a named or designated doctor or nurse
- If acute sexual abuse is a concern, undertake an initial inspection to ensure there is no serious bleeding requiring immediate action, then liaise with seniors to plan a joint forensic examination

Referral to social services

- If you consider the child may be a 'child in need' or 'at risk of suffering significant harm' you must follow local and national child protection procedures and refer the child and family to children's social care. Always inform your seniors, preferably in advance, but do not delay protecting a child you think may be at risk
- Try to discuss any concerns with the child, appropriate to their age and understanding, but their lack of agreement does not prohibit referral
- You should generally tell the parent you are referring to social services (unless this may place the child at greater risk, especially in intrafamilial sexual abuse) but this will be difficult and distressing so ensure you are prepared and suitably supported
- If the child is already known to social services, inform the allocated social worker
- Follow up any verbal referral in writing as soon as possible and always within 48 hours

In an emergency

Police and the NSPCC have legal powers to intervene to take a child to a 'place of safety'. If a parent removes a child before you are satisfied they are safe, any police officer can be called to prevent them or recover the child (social services would then be involved).

Pitfalls in diagnosis

- Mongolian blue spot – on buttocks and back of babies, may rarely be seen on any part of the body
- Recent viral infection, especially erythema infectiosum (parvovirus, causing 'slapped cheek disease')
- Clotting disorders, congenital or following infection, medication or blood dyscrasia
- Accidental or organic causes where the history and presentation has become garbled between multiple caregivers, e.g. nursery, grandparents, babysitters
- Bony abnormalities on X-ray that turn out to be normal variants

TOP TIPS

- Always consider child abuse as a possible differential diagnosis
- Believe what you see and make sure the explanation fits you findings
- Work with the family but keep the child's experience firmly in focus
- Babies under 1 year are most at risk of severe injury and death from abuse
- Always take bruising in a non-mobile child very seriously
- Review the number of times the child has presented to healthcare workers
- When in doubt get a senior opinion

Reference

DFES (Department for Education) (2006) *What to Do if You're Worried a Child is being Abused*. http://www.education.gov.uk/publications/standard/publicationdetail/page1/dfes-04320-2006 (last accessed 20 May 2013).

Figure 61.1 Signs of specific illnesses

Diagnosis to be considered	Symptoms and signs in conjunction with fever	Diagnosis to be considered	Symptoms and signs in conjunction with fever
Meningococcal disease	• Non-blanching rash, particularly with one or more of the following: – an ill-looking child – lesions larger than 2 mm in diameter (purpura) – capillary refill time of ≥3 seconds – neck stiffness	Urinary tract infection	• Vomiting • Poor feeding • Lethargy • Irritability • Abdominal pain or tenderness • Urinary frequency or dysuria • Offensive urine or haematuria
Meningitis	• Neck stiffness • Bulging fontanelle • Decreased level of consciousness • Convulsive status epilepticus	Septic arthritis	• Swelling of a limb or joint • Not using an extremity • Non-weight-bearing
Herpes simplex encephalitis	• Focal neurological signs • Focal seizures • Decreased level of consciousness	Kawasaki disease	• Fever for more than 5 days and at least four of the following: – bilateral conjunctival injection – change in mucous membranes – change in the extremities – polymorphous rash – cervical lymphadenopathy
Pneumonia	• Tachypnoea (RR: age 0–5 months >60 breaths/min; age 6–12 months >50 breaths/min; age >12 months>40 breaths/min) • Crackles • Nasal flaring • Chest indrawing • Cyanosis • Oxygen saturation ≤95%		

Figure 61.2 Traffic light system for the febrile child

	Green: low risk	Amber: intermediate risk	Red: high risk
Colour	Normal colour skin, lips and tongue	Parent/carer reports pallor	Pale/mottled/ashen/blue
Activity	• Responds normally to social cues • Content/smiles • Stays awake or awakens quickly • Strong normal cry/not crying	• Not responding normally to social cues • Wakes only with prolonged stimulation • Decreased activity • No smile	• No response to social cues • Appears ill to a healthcare professional • Unable to rouse or if roused does not stay awake • Weak, high-pitched or continuous cry
Respiration		• Nasal flaring • Tachypnoea:RR >50 breaths/min age 6–12 months; >40 breaths/min age >12 months • Oxygen saturation ≤95% in air • Crackles	• Grunting • Tachypnoea RR >60 breaths/min • Moderate or severe chest indrawing
Hydration	• Normal skin and eyes • Moist mucous membranes	• Dry mucous membrane • Poor feeding in infants • CRT 3 seconds or more • Reduced urine output	• Reduced skin turgor
Other	• None of the amber or red symptoms or signs	• Fever for 5 days or more • Swollen limb or joint • Not weight-bearing/not using extremity • A new lump >2 cm	• Age 0–3 months: temp 38°C or more • Age 3–6 months: temp 39°C or more • Non-blanching rash • Neck stiffness • Bulging fontanelle • Status epilepticus • Focal neurological signs • Focal seizures • Bile-stained vomiting

Few things worry parents more than a high temperature in a child and it is a common prompt to seek medical advice. This chapter covers the major causes and management of the condition.

Fever is a non-specific sign, and its cause is usually a self-limiting viral infection, but despite no evidence of a clear source in the early stages, fever may be an early sign of a significant or life-threatening infection (Fig. 61.1).

Infection remains the most frequent cause of death in children under 5. Following guidelines (NICE Guideline 47) will reduce the risk of missing a seriously ill child at a treatable stage. Good, culturally appropriate communication between the doctor and parents or carers of children with fever is essential, supported by written information.

Detection of fever

Note that oral and rectal routes should not routinely be used to measure the body temperature of children aged 0–5 years.

- In infants under the age of 4 weeks, body temperature should be measured with an electronic thermometer in the axilla
- In children aged 4 weeks to 5 years use an electronic thermometer or a chemical dot thermometer in the axilla, or an infrared tympanic thermometer
- If parents report the child has a fever this should be taken seriously

Assessment

- First identify whether any immediately life-threatening features are present, including compromised airway, breathing or circulation, or decreased level of consciousness
- Assess the child for the presence or absence of risk factors for serious illness using the traffic light system (Fig. 61.2).
- Measure temperature, heart rate, respiratory rate and capillary refill time as part of the routine assessment of a febrile child

Remote assessment, e.g. telephone

Children with **ANY** 'red' features who do not seem to have an immediately life-threatening illness should be urgently assessed by a doctor in a face-to-face setting within 2 hours.

Assessment by the non-paediatric practitioner, e.g. GP

If **ANY** 'amber' features are present and no diagnosis has been reached, refer to specialist paediatric care for further assessment **or** give parents a 'safety net' of one or more of the following:

- Provide verbal and/or written information on warning symptoms and how further healthcare can be accessed (ensure they can read and understand the information)
- Arrange follow up at a specified time and place
- Liaise with others, including the out-of-hours doctor, to ensure direct access for the child if further assessment is required

Note that oral antibiotics should **NOT** be prescribed to children with fever without an apparent source. Antipyretic agents do not prevent febrile convulsions and should not be used specifically for this purpose.

Assessment by the paediatric specialist service

- Infants younger than 3 months with fever should be observed and have vital signs measured (temperature, heart rate, respiratory rate)
- Children with fever without an apparent source presenting with one or more 'red' features should have investigations performed:
  - Full blood count
  - Blood culture
  - C-reactive protein
  - Urine testing for urinary tract infection
- Consider further investigations in children with 'red' features, as guided by clinical assessment:
  - Lumbar puncture in children of all ages (if not contraindicated)
  - Chest X-ray irrespective of temperature and white blood cell count
  - Serum electrolytes
  - Blood gases

Further clinical assessment of the child with fever

Children with feverish illness should be assessed using the traffic light system (Fig. 61.2):

- Children with **ANY** 'red' symptoms or signs should be recognized as being in a high-risk group for serious illness

- Children with **ANY** 'amber' symptoms should be recognized as being in at least an intermediate-risk group for serious illness
- Children who have **ALL** of the 'green' features, and **NONE** of the 'red' or 'amber' risk features, should be recognized as being in a low-risk group for serious illness

Measure temperature, heart rate, respiratory rate and capillary refill time as part of the routine assessment of a febrile child

- A raised heart rate can be a sign of serious illness, e.g. septic shock
- A capillary refill time of 3 seconds or longer is an 'amber' sign
- Measure BP if the heart rate or capillary refill time is abnormal
- Height or duration of temperature alone do not identify children with serious illness. However, high-risk groups for serious illness are:
  - Children younger than 3 months with a temperature of 38°C
  - Children aged 3–6 months with a temperature of 39°C or higher
- Assess for signs of dehydration by looking for: prolonged capillary refill time, abnormal skin turgor, abnormal respiratory pattern, weak pulse, cool extremities

Symptoms and signs of specific illnesses

Look for a source of fever and check for the presence of symptoms and signs that are associated with specific diseases (Fig. 61.1). Remember to enquire about recent travel abroad and consider the possibility of imported infections depending on the region visited.

Meningococcal disease or meningitis should be considered in any child with fever, **with or without** a non-blanching rash, if **ANY** of the following features are present: an ill-looking child, purpura larger than 2 mm in diameter, capillary refill time (CRT) of 3 seconds or longer, neck stiffness, bulging fontanelle, decreased level of consciousness, convulsive status epilepticus

Note that the classic signs of meningitis (neck stiffness, bulging fontanelle, high-pitched cry) are often absent in infants with bacterial meningitis.

Herpes simplex encephalitis may present with fever and **ANY** of: focal neurological signs, focal seizures or a decreased level of consciousness.

Pneumonia may present with fever and **ANY** of: tachypnoea, chest crackles, nasal flaring, chest indrawing, cyanosis or oxygen saturation of 95% or less in air.

Urinary tract infection may present in **ANY** child younger than 3 months with fever; **OR** in a child aged 3 months and older with fever **AND** one or more of: vomiting, poor feeding, lethargy, irritability, abdominal pain or tenderness, urinary frequency or dysuria, offensive urine or haematuria.

Septic arthritis/osteomyelitis may present with fever and **ANY** of: limb or joint swelling, not using an extremity or non-weight bearing.

Kawasaki disease may present with fever lasting over 5 days **AND** with four of the following five (rarely, incomplete/atypical Kawasaki disease may be diagnosed with fewer): bilateral conjunctival injection, changed upper respiratory mucous membranes (e.g. injected pharynx, cracked lips, strawberry tongue), oedema, erythema or desquamation of extremities, polymorphous rash or cervical lymphadenopathy.

TOP TIPS

- Get as accurate a temperature reading as you can
- Consider the state of arousal of the child
- If in doubt, admit it
- Use the traffic lights system
- Call for experienced help
- Keep parents fully informed of what you are doing

Figure 62.1 Features likely to be asthma

- Frequent, recurrent cough, wheeze, breathing difficulty or chest tightness
- Worse at night or early morning
- Occurs apart from URTI
- Triggered by cold/damp air, pets, laughter, emotion, exercise, etc.
- History of atopy
- Family history of atopy or asthma
- Widespread wheeze on auscultation
- Improved symptoms/lung function with treatment

Figure 62.2 Features not likely to be asthma

- Symptoms only with URTI, no interval symptoms
- Cough, but no wheeze or breathing difficulty
- History of moist cough
- Feel dizzy, light-headed, peripheral tingling
- Repeatedly normal chest exam during symptoms
- Normal PEFR during symptoms
- No response to trial of therapy
- Indicators of alternative diagnosis

Figure 62.3 Other causes of cough in childhood

- Pertussis
- Passive smoking
- Allergic rhinitis
- Catarrh, sinusitis and post nasal drip
- Gastro-oesophageal reflux
- Post-viral hyperresponsive airways
- Inhaled foreign body
- Congenital heart disease
- Congenital malformation
- Tuberculosis

Figure 62.4 Summary of stepwise management of asthma in children

(a) Less than 5 years

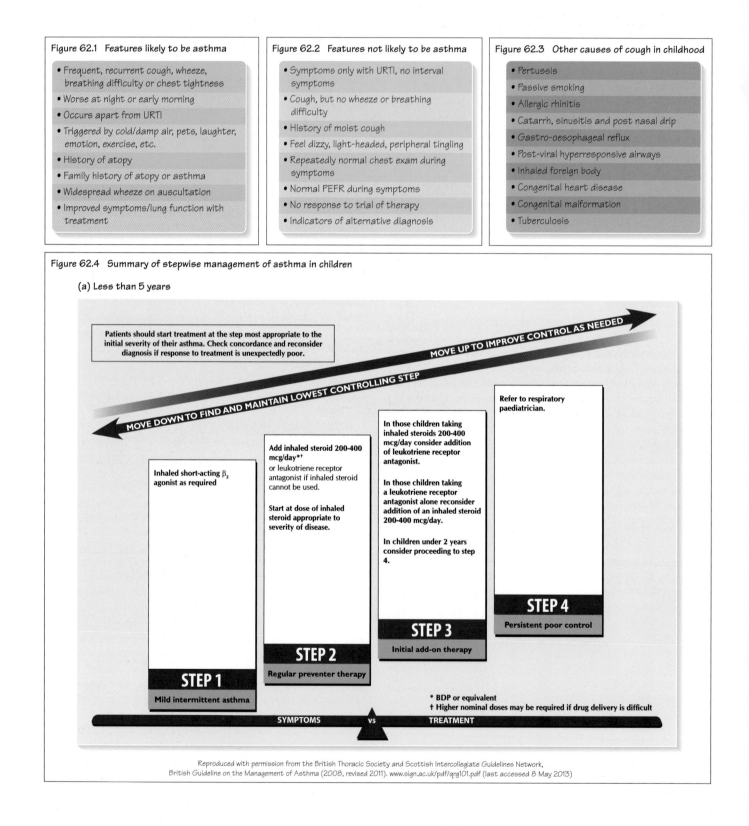

Patients should start treatment at the step most appropriate to the initial severity of their asthma. Check concordance and reconsider diagnosis if response to treatment is unexpectedly poor.

MOVE UP TO IMPROVE CONTROL AS NEEDED

MOVE DOWN TO FIND AND MAINTAIN LOWEST CONTROLLING STEP

Inhaled short-acting β_2 agonist as required

STEP 1
Mild intermittent asthma

Add inhaled steroid 200–400 mcg/day*† or leukotriene receptor antagonist if inhaled steroid cannot be used.

Start at dose of inhaled steroid appropriate to severity of disease.

STEP 2
Regular preventer therapy

In those children taking inhaled steroids 200–400 mcg/day consider addition of leukotriene receptor antagonist.

In those children taking a leukotriene receptor antagonist alone reconsider addition of an inhaled steroid 200–400 mcg/day.

In children under 2 years consider proceeding to step 4.

STEP 3
Initial add-on therapy

Refer to respiratory paediatrician.

STEP 4
Persistent poor control

* BDP or equivalent
† Higher nominal doses may be required if drug delivery is difficult

SYMPTOMS   vs   TREATMENT

Reproduced with permission from the British Thoracic Society and Scottish Intercollegiate Guidelines Network, British Guideline on the Management of Asthma (2008, revised 2011). www.sign.ac.uk/pdf/qrg101.pdf (last accessed 8 May 2013)

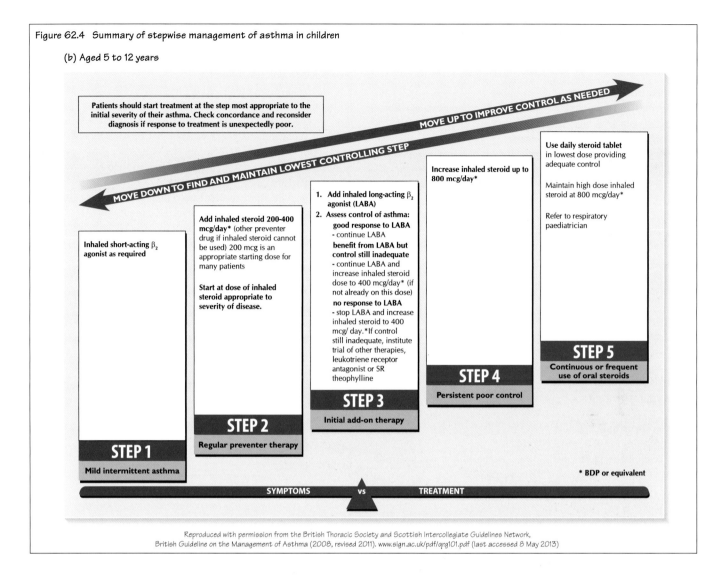

Figure 62.4 Summary of stepwise management of asthma in children

(b) Aged 5 to 12 years

Patients should start treatment at the step most appropriate to the initial severity of their asthma. Check concordance and reconsider diagnosis if response to treatment is unexpectedly poor.

MOVE UP TO IMPROVE CONTROL AS NEEDED

MOVE DOWN TO FIND AND MAINTAIN LOWEST CONTROLLING STEP

Inhaled short-acting β₂ agonist as required

Add inhaled steroid 200-400 mcg/day* (other preventer drug if inhaled steroid cannot be used) 200 mcg is an appropriate starting dose for many patients

Start at dose of inhaled steroid appropriate to severity of disease.

1. Add inhaled long-acting β₂ agonist (LABA)
2. Assess control of asthma:
   good response to LABA
   - continue LABA
   benefit from LABA but control still inadequate
   - continue LABA and increase inhaled steroid dose to 400 mcg/day* (if not already on this dose)
   no response to LABA
   - stop LABA and increase inhaled steroid to 400 mcg/ day.*If control still inadequate, institute trial of other therapies, leukotriene receptor antagonist or SR theophylline

Increase inhaled steroid up to 800 mcg/day*

Use daily steroid tablet in lowest dose providing adequate control

Maintain high dose inhaled steroid at 800 mcg/day*

Refer to respiratory paediatrician

STEP 1
Mild intermittent asthma

STEP 2
Regular preventer therapy

STEP 3
Initial add-on therapy

STEP 4
Persistent poor control

STEP 5
Continuous or frequent use of oral steroids

* BDP or equivalent

SYMPTOMS vs TREATMENT

Reproduced with permission from the British Thoracic Society and Scottish Intercollegiate Guidelines Network, British Guideline on the Management of Asthma (2008, revised 2011). www.sign.ac.uk/pdf/qrg101.pdf (last accessed 8 May 2013)

Breathing problems in children are common but like all childhood illnesses are a great deal of concern to parents. This chapter covers the differential diagnosis and management of those with asthma.

Is it asthma?

Cough, wheeze and difficulty breathing at the time of upper respiratory tract infection (URTI) is extremely common in children (30% of under 3 year olds). This is partly due to simple physics (Poiseuille's law) – flow is proportional to the 4th power of the radius of a tube. Thus slight narrowing of an airway with mucus will considerably reduce flow, causing wheeze. This may represent a local inflammatory process, but not the reversible bronchospasm of asthma.

Asthma (chronic reversible bronchospasm with inflammation) can be difficult to diagnose in children. It is essentially a clinical diagnosis of the characteristic pattern of episodic symptoms in the absence of an alternative cause. It can be particularly difficult to diagnose in the under fives, where spirometry is not possible. This may be managed by either watchful waiting or a trial of treatment, and review.

Initial assessment

- Child has cough, wheeze, difficulty breathing or chest tightness
- Look for key features in history and examination (Fig. 62.1)

- Consider alternatives to exclude other diagnoses (Figs 62.2 and 62.3)
- Assess and record reasons for deciding whether child has a high, intermediate or low probability of asthma

For a child with a high probability of asthma

- Note the criteria, and start a trial of treatment
- Review and assess response
- Reserve further testing for those with a poor response

For a child with a low probability of asthma

- Note the absence of criteria for asthma
- Consider referral and further investigation of symptoms (Fig. 62.4)

For a child with an intermediate probability of asthma

- Note the criteria and assess PEFR or FEV₁ if possible
- If unable to assess PEFR, initiate a treatment trial for a fixed time
- Assess reversibility with a trial of inhaled bronchodilator
- If no response, consider investigation of alternative diagnoses
- Treat as asthma if there is significant improvement with treatment
- Use minimum effective dose; review later to reduce or stop

Managing acute asthma in children

Assess the severity of the event: life-threatening or acute severe attacks require urgent hospital admission.

Children under 2 years

• Assessment of young children can be difficult as intermittent wheezing may be seen with viral URTI, and response to anti-asthmatics is variable
• Differential diagnosis includes bronchiolitis, pneumonia, aspiration pneumonitis, tracheomalacia, complications of other conditions including congenital abnormalities, cystic fibrosis, prematurity and low birth weight
• Treat with inhaled β_2-agonists via a paediatric metered dose inhaler (pMDI), spacer and face mask. Oral β_2-agonists are not recommended
• Consider steroid treatment early (10 mg soluble prednisolone for up to 3 days)
• Consider adding inhaled ipratropium bromide to inhaled β_2-agonists in more severe cases

Children over 2 years

Life-threatening asthma

• $SPO_2 < 92\%$, PEFR < 33–50% of predicted
• Poor respiratory effort, cyanosed, exhausted
• Hypotension, falling heat rate
• Confusion, coma

Acute severe asthma

• $SPO_2 < 92\%$, PEFR 33–50% of predicted
• Can't complete sentence in one breath, too breathless to talk or feed
• Pulse > 125/min (5+ years) or 140/min (2–5 years)
• RR > 30/min (5+ years) or 40/min (2–5 years)

Management of acute attacks outside hospital

• Inhaled β_2-agonists – give 2 puffs every 2 minutes, up to 10 puffs
• If no improvement, refer to hospital. Keep giving inhaler during transit
• Use oxygen and nebulized β_2-agonists in the ambulance
• $SPO_2 < 92\%$ in air after initial bronchodilator use – child is likely to need intensive inpatient treatment
• Increasing tachycardia generally means worsening severity
• Note progress of breathing, wheeze and use of accessory muscles to breathe
• Note conscious level and any agitation. Give calm reassurance
• Remember that clinical signs do not always correlate well with severity, some children in severe attack may not appear distressed. Monitor vital signs

Management of acute attacks in hospital

• In life-threatening attacks or if $SPO_2 < 94\%$, give high-flow oxygen via a tight-fitting face mask or nasal prongs to normalize the SPO_2
• Treat with inhaled β_2-agonists via a pMDI and spacer (and face mask if needed)
• If poor response, add inhaled ipratropium bromide 250 μg to the nebulized β_2-agonists. Ipratropium bromide doses can be repeated

• If poor response to inhaled treatment, consider single IV bolus of salbutamol (15 μg/kg over 10 minutes)
• Discontinue long-acting β_2-agonists when short-acting β_2-agonists are required more than 4-hourly
• Use steroids early, usually 20 mg for 3 days (age 2–5 years) or 30–40 mg for 3 days (age > 5 years). If the dose is vomited, repeat the dose or consider IV dose. If already on steroids, use 2 mg/kg to a max. of 60 mg. Longer duration of treatment may be necessary. Weaning is needed for courses over 14 days
• Antibiotics should not be used unless clearly indicated by a diagnosed infection
• Aminophylline is not recommended in mild to moderate attacks but may be used in HDU/paediatric intensive care unit (PICU) for severe or life-threatening bronchospasm unresponsive to maximal doses of bronchodilators and steroids

Long-term management of stable asthma

• Any child admitted to hospital with acute exacerbation should have a hospital review within a month
• Children with asthma should be reviewed on a regular basis, ideally in a specialist GP-based asthma clinic, with patient PEFR monitoring
• Stepwise care allows an increase or reduction of long-term treatment depending on the level of symptom control (Fig. 62.4)
• Enquire specifically about exercise-induced asthma, limitation of activity, sleep problems and nocturnal cough, and modify treatment accordingly
• Metered dose inhalers should only be prescribed after patients have been trained in their use and have demonstrated good technique
• Children too young to use inhalers must be given medication through a spacer with face mask or nebulizer as required
• A range of administration methods is available (aerosol, dry powder) which can be used to improve control and adherence to treatment
• Avoidance of environmental allergens and triggers (especially cigarette smoke, house dust mite, damp, mould and animal dander) may be important factors in managing asthma long term
• Patient education and participation in long-term management of their condition, reduction of disease burden and improving quality of life

---

TOP TIPS

• Take a full history including family history and presence of pets in the house
• Check for associated allergies
• Keep parents informed at all times
• Know that nearly all care will be carried out in primary care
• Give parents supporting information to take away

Reference

BRS (British Thoracic Society) and SIGN (Scottish Intercollegiate Guidelines Network) (2009) *British Guideline on the Management of Asthma.* http://www.sign.ac.uk/pdf/qrg101.pdf (last accessed 8 May 2013).

Diarrhoea, vomiting and constipation in young children

Figure 63.1 The Bristol stool form scale

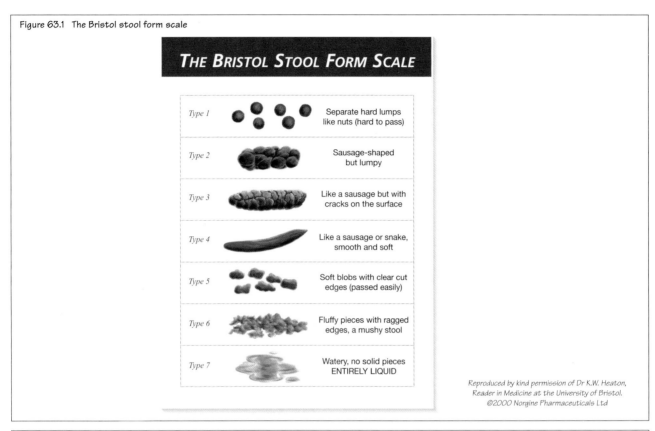

THE BRISTOL STOOL FORM SCALE

Type 1		Separate hard lumps like nuts (hard to pass)
Type 2		Sausage-shaped but lumpy
Type 3		Like a sausage but with cracks on the surface
Type 4		Like a sausage or snake, smooth and soft
Type 5		Soft blobs with clear cut edges (passed easily)
Type 6		Fluffy pieces with ragged edges, a mushy stool
Type 7		Watery, no solid pieces ENTIRELY LIQUID

Reproduced by kind permission of Dr K.W. Heaton,
Reader in Medicine at the University of Bristol.
©2000 Norgine Pharmaceuticals Ltd

Figure 63.2 Clinical features of dehydration and shock, with red flags

Increasing severity of dehydration →

	No clinically detectable dehydration	Clinical dehydration	Clinical shock
Symptoms (remote and face-to-face assessments)	Appears well	► Appears to be unwell or deteriorating	–
	Alert and responsive	► Altered responsiveness (e.g. irritable, lethargic)	Decreased level of consciousness
	Normal urine output	Decreased urine output	–
	Skin colour unchanged	Skin colour unchanged	Pale or mottled skin
	Warm extremities	Warm extremities	Cold extremities
Signs (face-to-face assessments)	Alert and responsive	► Altered responsiveness (e.g. irritable, lethargic)	Decreased level of consciousness
	Skin colour unchanged	Skin colour unchanged	Pale or mottled skin
	Warm extremities	Warm extremities	Cold extremities
	Eyes not sunken	► Sunken eyes	–
	Moist mucous membranes (except after a drink)	Dry mucous membranes (except for 'mouth breather')	–
	Normal heart rate	► Tachycardia	Tachycardia
	Normal breathing pattern	► Tachypnoea	Tachypnoea
	Normal peripheral pulses	Normal peripheral pulses	Weak peripheral pulses
	Normal capillary refill time	Normal capillary refill time	Prolonged capillary refill time
	Normal skin turgor	► Reduced skin turgor	–
	Normal blood pressure	Normal blood pressure	Hypotension (decompensation shock)

This chapter covers the management of diarrhoea, vomiting and constipation in the young child (Fig. 63.1).

Diarrhoea and vomiting (D&V)

Diarrhoea, with or without vomiting, is a common presentation of infective **gastroenteritis** in young children, usually caused by an enteric virus, and resolving spontaneously within a few days. Children may be brought for medical advice (16% of all presentations to one emergency department) if symptoms are severe. The medical task is to identify and manage complications such as **dehydration** or **hypernatraemia**, which can be life threatening, and to identify other rarer gastrointestinal or systemic illnesses presenting with D&V.

Diagnosis

Consider any of the following as possible indicators of diagnoses other than gastroenteritis:

- Fever – temperature of 38°C or more (age under 3 months) or 39°C or more (age 3+ months)
- Shortness of breath, tachypnoea
- Altered conscious state, neck stiffness, bulging fontanelle in infants
- Non-blanching rash (NB consider meningitis/septicaemia for all the above)
- Blood and/or mucus in stool (consider inflammatory bowel disease)
- Bilious (green) vomit, severe or localized abdominal pain, abdominal distension or rebound tenderness (consider obstruction or acute abdomen)

    Do a stool culture if:

- You suspect septicaemia
- There is blood and mucus in the stool (also beware of *Escherichia coli* 0157 and the risk of haemolytic uraemic syndrome)
- The child is known to be immunocompromised

    Consider a stool culture if there is diagnostic uncertainty, if diarrhoea is prolonged over 7 days, or the child has been abroad.

    Assess dehydration and shock (Fig. 63.2). Assess whether the child:

- Appears unwell, with altered responsiveness, or is irritable or lethargic
- Has decreased urine output
- Has pale or mottled skin or cold extremities

Children at greater risk of dehydration or recurrence

- Aged under 1 year, especially under 6 months
- Low birth weight, or malnourished babies
- More than five diarrhoeal stools or two vomits in the past 24 hours
- Children who have not received or tolerated extra fluids
- Infants who have stopped breastfeeding during the D&V

Fluid management

For the **primary prevention of dehydration** in children with gastroenteritis but without clinical dehydration:

- Continue breastfeeding and other milk feeds
- Encourage fluid intake (but not fruit juices and carbonated drinks)
- Offer oral rehydration solution (ORS) to high-risk children

Treatment of dehydration without shock

- Use low osmolarity ORS (240–250 mOsm/L) for rehydration, giving 50 mL/kg over 4 hours to replace fluid deficit, administered as frequent sips. Use an NG tube if unable to drink or persistent vomiting
- Monitor response to oral rehydration with regular clinical assessment

- A child with red flag features (Fig. 63.2) deteriorating clinically despite ORS, or persistently vomiting oral or NG ORS, will need IV rehydration
- For IV rehydration with no hypernatraemia, use isotonic fluids (normal saline ± 5% glucose) for fluid deficit replacement and maintenance. Add 50 mL/kg for fluid deficit replacement and maintenance, and monitor clinical response

Treatment of shock

IV fluids are required if shock is suspected or confirmed.

- Treat shock with a rapid IV infusion of 20 mL/kg of normal (0.9%) saline
- If shock persists after the first rapid IV infusion, repeat rapid IV 20 mL/kg of normal (0.9%) saline **and** consider possible causes other than dehydration. Consider involving a PICU specialist if shock persists after the second infusion
- Following initial rapid IV fluid boluses for shock, add 100 mL/kg fluid deficit replacement and maintenance, and monitor clinical response
- Measure electrolytes (plasma sodium, potassium, urea, creatinine, glucose) at outset, monitor regularly and adjust fluid replacement accordingly. IV potassium supplementation may be indicated once the plasma potassium level is known

Treatment of hypernatraemic dehydration

This complication can lead to serious consequences.

- Clinical features include jittery movements, increased muscle tone, hyperreflexia, convulsions, drowsiness or coma
- Blood testing for plasma sodium, potassium, urea, creatinine and glucose is indicated if clinical features suggest hypernatraemia
- Measure venous blood acid–base status and chloride concentration if shock is suspected or confirmed
- Use low osmolarity ORS (240–250 mOsm/L) for rehydration, including in hypernatraemia
- If IV fluid therapy is needed for hypernatraemic dehydration, get urgent expert advice on fluid management
- Use isotonic fluids (normal saline ± 5% glucose) for fluid deficit replacement and maintenance, replacing the fluid deficit slowly – typically over 48 hours
- Monitor plasma sodium frequently, aiming to reduce it at a rate of less than 0.5 mmol/L per hour
- Attempt early, gradual introduction of ORS during IV fluid therapy. If tolerated, stop IV fluids and complete rehydration orally

Fluid management after rehydration

- Encourage fluids, breastfeeding and other milk feeds
- Where there is increased risk of recurrent dehydration, offer 5 mL/kg of ORS after each large watery stool
- Do **NOT** use antidiarrhoeal medications

Antibiotic therapy in gastroenteritis

Antibiotics are indicated only for specific situations:

- Suspected or confirmed septicaemia
- Extraintestinal spread of bacterial infection
- *Salmonella* gastroenteritis if child is younger than 6 months or malnourished or immunocompromised
- *Clostridium difficile*-associated pseudomembranous enterocolitis, giardiasis, dysenteric shigellosis, dysenteric amoebiasis or cholera

- For children who have recently been abroad, seek specialist advice about antibiotic therapy

Constipation

Constipation is a common problem in childhood, with a prevalence of 5–20%, and a 33% chronicity rate. It may present as infrequent bowel motions, but also as overflow diarrhoea, soiling, abdominal pain, flatulence and wind, rectal pain or fissure, abdominal distension or pain, nausea, loss of appetite, withholding of stool, general malaise or irritability. Chronic constipation can also impact on urinary continence and UTI, constipation sometimes presenting with daytime wetting, especially in girls.

Children – like adults – have varying bowel transit times, but individuals tend to be consistent through their life course, and may be habitually constipated unless they take steps to manage their bowels.

Assessment and diagnosis

History and examination should identify any 'red flag' or treatable causes, allow a firm diagnosis of idiopathic constipation, and help plan appropriate management. Investigations for thyroid function and to exclude cystic fibrosis may be required. Investigations such as abdominal X-ray, ultrasound, endoscopy or manometry are not indicated. Digital rectal examination or biopsy should only be undertaken in a specialist setting.

Red flags: if any 'red flag' features are present, then further paediatric assessment is needed. It is not advisable to start treatment for constipation until a firm diagnosis is reached.
- Constipation from birth or first few weeks of life, including a 48-hour delay in passing meconium at birth or ribbon stools – consider Hirschprung's disease (atonic segment)
- Previously undiagnosed leg weakness, motor delay or urinary symptoms – consider spinal cord compression or abnormality
- Abdominal distension or vomiting – consider obstruction (e.g. volvulus, intussusception)
- Developmental delay or abnormal reflexes □ consider hypothyroidism

- Faltering growth or chest infections – consider cystic fibrosis, coeliac disease, immune disorder, hypercalcaemia, diabetes insipidus
- Concern about child abuse (such as neglect, underfeeding, faltering growth, sexual abuse)

Management of idiopathic constipation

- Advise on increasing fluids and fibre in the diet, and bowel habit hygiene, especially responding promptly to the 'call to stool'
- Use a macrogol laxative in the first instance, in sufficient doses (up to 8 sachets/day to correct fecal impaction, reduced to a maintenance dose following a response)
- Add in a stimulant laxative if necessary (picosulfate or bisacodyl)
- Maintenance medication may need to be used long term in doses higher than those recommended by the BNF – discuss with parents and gain informed consent to this 'off label' prescribing

---

TOP TIPS

- Take a full history including diet and medication
- Assess the child's state of hydration at presentation
- Children can dehydrate quickly so reassess early
- If child is alert always try oral rehydration first
- Investigate the primary cause with cultures and blood tests
- Keep parents informed at all times

References

National Institute for Health and Care Excellence (NICE) (2009) *Management of Acute Diarrhoea and Vomiting due to Gastoenteritis in Children under 5*. Clinical Guideline 84. http://www.nice.org.uk/CG84 (last accessed 20 May 2013).

National Institute for Health and Care Excellence (NICE) (2010) *Constipation in Children and Young People*. Clinical Guideline 99. http://guidance.nice.org.uk/CG99/NICEGuidance/doc/English (last accessed 20 May 2013).

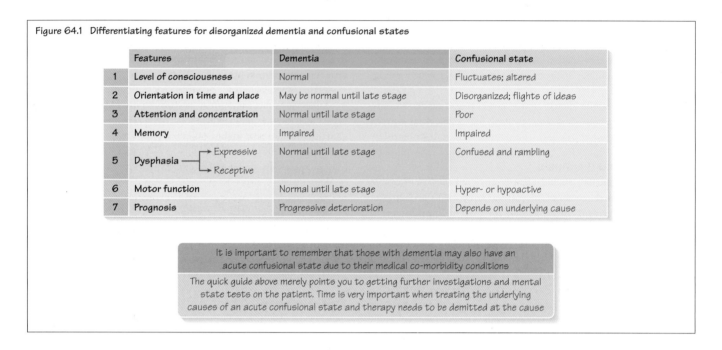

Figure 64.1 Differentiating features for disorganized dementia and confusional states

	Features	Dementia	Confusional state
1	Level of consciousness	Normal	Fluctuates; altered
2	Orientation in time and place	May be normal until late stage	Disorganized; flights of ideas
3	Attention and concentration	Normal until late stage	Poor
4	Memory	Impaired	Impaired
5	Dysphasia → Expressive / Receptive	Normal until late stage	Confused and rambling
6	Motor function	Normal until late stage	Hyper- or hypoactive
7	Prognosis	Progressive deterioration	Depends on underlying cause

It is important to remember that those with dementia may also have an acute confusional state due to their medical co-morbidity conditions

The quick guide above merely points you to getting further investigations and mental state tests on the patient. Time is very important when treating the underlying causes of an acute confusional state and therapy needs to be demitted at the cause

This chapter covers the issues of confusional states in the elderly. It is important to be able to differentiate a treatable confusional state from dementia. The history and onset of the episode is therefore crucial as is a discussion with relatives or carers of the patient.

Delirium

This affects about 20% of the elderly in hospital and is defined as an acute confusional state. It can manifest itself in several ways:
- Cognitive impairment (principally inattention)
- Altered state of arousal
- Disrupted sleep patterns
- Hallucinations
- Delusions
- Drowsiness

It is important to remember that delirium is a reaction to an acute event. Your history, examination and investigation should be geared to uncovering the root cause. In the elderly the cause may be multifactorial due to co-morbidities, and a simple urinary tract infection or chest infection can be enough to tip them into a state of delirium. Consider the following:
- Any acute illness
- Current drug treatment or alteration to therapy
- Alcohol consumption or withdrawal
- Sugar or electrolyte disturbance
- Relapse of a chronic condition

Your investigations should therefore focus on any alteration to drug therapy, history of drug or alcohol misuse and the following screens:
- Blood sugar
- FBC and ESR
- Urea and electrolytes
- Urinalysis
- Blood cultures
- Chest X-ray
- Oxygen saturation
- Lumbar puncture
- MRI scan if no other cause is found

The frequency with which delirium occurs in the elderly in the hospital setting suggests that you should consider all elderly admissions at risk and be proactive in minimizing the risks. Hearing and sight impairment need to be considered as does their nutritional state (which may not improve in hospital). Undertake a mini mental state examination (Fig. 64.1). Always check medication or changes to medication. Speak to relatives or carers about the patient's normal demeanour.

Treatment should be based on the root cause of the delirium.

Dementia

Dementia is a catch all phrase to describe a group of diseases that affect the brain. It leads to a progressive loss of brain cells and therefore gets progressively worse over time. You will come across an increasing number of patients with signs and symptoms of dementia as well as their presenting acute illnesses.

Symptoms
- Memory loss
- Behavioural changes
- Mood swings
- Inability to concentrate
- Difficulty in verbal expression and understanding
- Poor sense of time and place

Risk factors

Age remains the most significant risk factor with one in 50 people between the ages of 65 and 70 having some form of dementia compared with one in five people over 80 years. The reasons are not clear but may well relate to co-morbidities, e.g. high blood pressure, heart disease and stroke. Vascular dementia resulting from these diseases is more common in men than women. Alzheimer's (the commonest form of dementia) is, however, more common in women than in men.

Other risk factors fall into three main groups:

1 Genetic – this is more usual in families where the disease appears earlier in life, e.g. Huntington's disease, familial Alzheimer's and the rare Niemann–Pick type C disease.

2 Co-morbidities – multiple sclerosis, Down's syndrome and HIV all increase the risk of developing dementia. Repeated head injury also increases the risk.

3 Lifestyle – diet is important in reducing the risk of the co-morbidities that increase the risk of dementia, such as smoking and excess alcohol consumption over many years. Regular physical activity also reduces the likelihood of vascular dementia by promoting a healthy cardiovascular system.

Diagnosis

The diagnosis can be particularly difficult in the early stages and referral to a specialist consultant can be important.

It is important to get a clear history from people close to the patient. A full examination including memory tests and a brain scan may be indicated. The mini mental state examination (Fig. 64.1) is the commonest tool for those with memory problems when considering a diagnosis of dementia.

Following the diagnosis, the patient should be followed up by a specialist who will be able to ensure that the necessary support is available for the patient and family. You may also want to put them in touch with the Alzheimer's Society (e-mail: enquiries@alzheimers.org.uk) who have a great deal of literature and help available for patients and carers.

Treatment

If there is a strong family history of dementia, in particular more than one family member with early-onset dementia, then you should refer the patient to a regional clinical genetics department. At these centres the patient or family member can be given the appropriate counselling as to whether they should proceed to have a test. It is clearly not straightforward as without a treatment that can repair a genetic defect the patient is only finding out a predictive assessment of developing the disease. Expert guidance is therefore required.

Since there are no current ways to cure the disease the mainstay of treatment is support to the patient and carers. There are drugs that can help the symptoms, particularly in the early stages.

There are two main types of medication used:

- Cholinesterase inhibitors (e.g. Aricept, Exelon and Reminyl)
- N-methyl-D-aspartate (NMDA) receptor antagonists (e.g. Ebixa)

The National Institute for Health and Care Excellence (NICE) recommends Aricept, Exelon and Reminyl for mild to moderate Alzheimer's and Ebixa for moderate to severe disease.

TOP TIPS

- Altered mental state in the elderly can be multisystem disease
- Always do a mini mental state examination
- Do a full examination and investigations for treatable causes
- Get a clear history from carers if possible
- Refer for specialist opinion

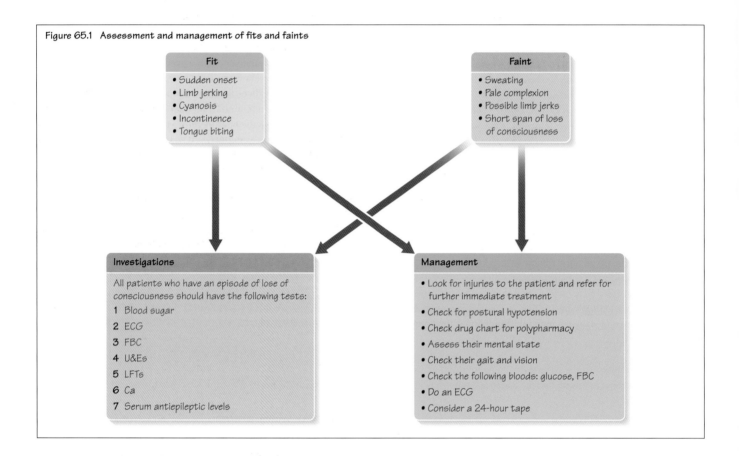

Figure 65.1 Assessment and management of fits and faints

Fit
- Sudden onset
- Limb jerking
- Cyanosis
- Incontinence
- Tongue biting

Faint
- Sweating
- Pale complexion
- Possible limb jerks
- Short span of loss of consciousness

Investigations

All patients who have an episode of lose of consciousness should have the following tests:
1 Blood sugar
2 ECG
3 FBC
4 U&Es
5 LFTs
6 Ca
7 Serum antiepileptic levels

Management
- Look for injuries to the patient and refer for further immediate treatment
- Check for postural hypotension
- Check drug chart for polypharmacy
- Assess their mental state
- Check their gait and vision
- Check the following bloods: glucose, FBC
- Do an ECG
- Consider a 24-hour tape

This chapter covers the immediate management and assessment of patients who have a fit or a faint. Remember they may also injure themselves by falling to the floor due to the fit or faint.

Fits, faints and falls are all common occurrences and you will be called to many episodes of these over your career. It is worth remembering that when you first see the patient you should remember the basic drill for those with an altered state of consciousness.

Check
- Airway
- Breathing
- Circulation
- Level of consciousness

Place in the recovery position as appropriate.

History
Once this has been quickly done it may be possible for you to get a **history** either from the patient or those present at the time of the incident. It is worth grouping fits and faints together as the distinction is not important for the immediate management of the case. Falls, particularly in the elderly, will be dealt with as separate events, though remember they too can faint and have fits.

When considering fits and faints remember the presentations in Fig. 65.1. This may be all you can ascertain from those present. Further history should then be taken from the patient when they are able and should include:
- Previous history
- Current medication
- Alcohol or drug ingestion
- Precipitating factors if known
- Time of day or night commonly for episode
- Nausea
- Hyperventilation
- Light headedness
- Co-morbidities, e.g. parkinsonism, diabetes
- Palpitations or chest pain

The essential element of the history is first to differentiate between the causes but also to find the root cause of the problem. The wrong management can have a profound effect on the lifestyle of a patient if a simple faint was investigated and treated as if it were epilepsy.

It is also important to ensure that anyone who has a definite seizure should have an MRI scan (or CT scan) looking for any intracranial lesions.

Treatment in fits and faints

A simple faint requires no treatment as the patient will regain consciousness fairly quickly. You need to ensure that they are in a safe environment while they fully recover their faculties.

In a fit the following should be tried for seizure control:

- Lorazepam 2 mg IV
- Diazepam 10 mg PR if you cannot get IV access

(Remember these doses are different in the young and elderly!) **IF THIS DOES NOT CONTROL THE FIT THEN YOU WILL REQUIRE SENIOR ASSISTANCE.**

- IV phenytoin should then be administered or sodium valproate if the patient is already on phenytoin as a routine medication

Status epilepticus is when a fit lasts longer than 30 minutes. This is a medical emergency with a high mortality. It is essential to find out the cause of the status and treat this to ensure a satisfactory outcome. Poor compliance, alcohol or drug misuse or infection are the common causes. Referral to intensive care and consideration of ventilation and anaesthesia are essential.

For the management of fits and faints, see Fig. 65.1.

Implications of a diagnosis of epilepsy

The diagnosis of epilepsy has a profound effect on the patient and their lifestyle. It may prevent them from continuing their current employment and driving a car. It is therefore important that the patient is kept fully informed of what the restrictions on their day-to-day activities are and what medication they need to take. This is specialist knowledge and therefore a referral to the appropriate clinic in the hospital is required.

Prevention of falls

There are many reasons why patients fall and since it is possible to prevent this happening in a large percentage of cases it is worth fully investigating. The following all need considering:

- Previous mobility (check their footwear)
- Current health
- Polypharmacy
- Eyesight
- Dementia

The cause may be obvious if related to a current illness like parkinsonism, hypotensive medication or nitrates that have caused the patient to momentarily collapse. Other causes may be less obvious and require further investigation, e.g. palpitations or vertebrobasilar insufficiency.

Next steps

The management of the patient is:

1 Deal with the immediate consequences of the fall
2 Investigate the cause of the fall (Fig. 65.1)
3 Reduce future episodes

The follow up of these patients is invariably multidisciplinary. The patient may need to be seen by a neurologist, physiotherapist, occupational therapist and a care of the elderly consultant and team. The patient may suffer a crisis of confidence having fallen over and this can be very difficult to treat. It may lead to isolation at home, not wanting to go out and ultimately depression. It is therefore essential that individuals are properly investigated and given appropriate follow up in the community. A visit to the patient's house may reveal that the furniture is tightly packed together and is easy to trip over, or that there is no hand rails for the stairs. Simple adjustments can have a marked effect on the number of falls and admissions to hospital that these patients receive.

You also need to remember that the medication you have prescribed can be the trigger for the falls. Think carefully about the effects the following drugs may have on the lifestyle of patients when they are out of the controlled, safe environment of a hospital ward:

- Benzodiazepines
- Antidepressants
- Hypertensive medication
- Diuretics and laxatives (and rushing to an upstairs toilet)

It is also worth thinking through what other drugs the patient may be taking at home in the form of pain relief and alcohol that may also lower their mental state.

TOP TIPS

- Fits need full investigation
- Review all medication for the causes of fits, faints and falls
- Involve the multidisciplinary team
- Ensure the patient understands fully what has happened
- Speak to carers and relatives about the management on discharge

Index

Note: page numbers in *italics* refer to figures, those in **bold** refer to tables.

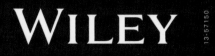

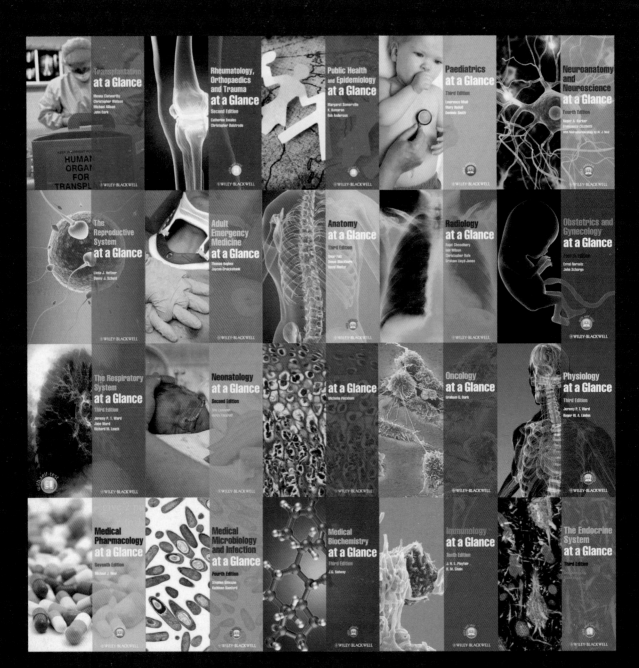

The at a Glance series

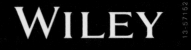